REMEMBERING SAM

Remembering Sam

The Life and Times of
SAM GALBRAITH

Managing Editor
GRAHAM TEASDALE
Literary Editor
BRIAN WILSON
with
NICOLA TENNANT
HARRY BURNS
ALISTAIR DARLING
DAVID HAMILTON

EDINBURGH

First published in 2016 by Birlinn Ltd
West Newington House
10 Newington Road
Edinburgh
EH9 1QS

www.birlinn.co.uk

ISBN: 978-1-78027-338-9

British Library Cataloguing in Publication Data
A catalogue record for this book is available from the British
Library

Typeset in Adobe Garamond Pro at Birlinn

Printed and bound by Grafica Veneta
www.graficaveneta.com

Contents

Contents

Illustrations

The Galbraith family on holiday at Ostel Bay, Kilbride, Argyll, August 1959.

In the mountains: Ben Nevis, 1970.

'Happy Days', Sam and Nicola in Val d'Illiez, Valais, Switzerland, 1981.

'Hitting the wall' at the Glasgow marathon, 1982.

Speaking from the health care workers' campaign bus, George Square, Glasgow, 1982.

'Oh, my big hobnailers', Leckelm, Ullapool, 1985.

Consultant Neurosurgeon, Institute of Neurological Sciences, Southern General Hospital, Glasgow, 1987.

Return to Westminster *en famille*, July 1990.

Sam and Jonathan Butler with three junior canvassers and the venerable Butler Land Rover, 1997.

Sam, Brian Wilson and Donald Dewar: New Ministers in the Scottish Office, May 1997.

'There shall be a Scottish Parliament', Edinburgh, 1 July 1999.

'Checking out the Chamber' of the Scottish Parliament on the Mound, Edinburgh, 30 June 1999.

Barbecue on the beach at Little Bernera, Lewis, with the Wilsons, Darlings and friends, 2000.

In front of *The City of Adelaide*, Irvine, the Scottish Maritime Museum, 2012.

Nicola, Sam, Heather, Mhairi and Fiona, January 2013.

Preface

The widespread sadness at the death of Sam Galbraith in August 2014 was accompanied by the wish that his remarkable personality and exceptional achievements should be captured in some lasting celebration of his life. Articles in medical journals and newspapers have charted his career as both an eminent doctor and a notable politician, but not the character behind the achievements. It is the purpose of this book to bring all these elements together.

To tell the story of Sam's life and times, based on personal experience, is beyond the capacity of any individual. Instead, this book draws on many different and complementary perspectives. Extracts from his speeches and writings let Sam speak for himself. The recollections of shared experiences, activities and achievements, enhanced by insights into his character and talents, have come together to create a portrait of the complex, distinctive person that Sam was.

The chapters are in a loose historical order, covering and linking the successive phases in Sam's life. They deal, with humour and honesty, with his early life in Greenock, his medical studies at Glasgow University, where he was the outstanding graduate of his year, and his rapid rise in neurosurgery, when he made fundamental advances in treating brain injuries and successfully undertook the most demanding kinds of surgery. They tell how his intense socialist principles, and a wish to make a difference on a wider scale, increasingly drew him to politics through the Labour Party, and to election as Member of Parliament in 1987.

Sam's lung transplantation just two years after becoming an MP left him with limited health. Despite this, he went on to hold ministerial posts first at Westminster, and then in the new Scottish Parliament. In government, he abolished markets in the NHS in Scotland, creating its enduring, co-ordinated, coherent system of care. He led the way in highlighting the relationship between deprivation and ill health which, to an astonishing extent, had hitherto been denied. In every aspect of his career Sam really made a lasting difference. After leaving Parliament he continued to put his talents to use in a range of public and voluntary roles.

The elements of Sam's character which these chapters convey include intelligence, vision, commitment, humour, irreverence, enjoyment of debate, of the outdoors, of Scottish culture and tradition and fun. Underlying all of these was a deep integrity, loyalty, selflessness and courage. They also affirm the importance to Sam of his family, first and foremost – Nicola, his wife, and their three daughters, Mhairi, Heather and Fiona, the eldest of whom was born only a few weeks before his transplant.

Reading these memories makes it easy to understand why Sam Galbraith was unique and inspired such respect and great affection; how much he contributed and how much he will continue to be missed.

The Galbraith Editorial Group: *Graham Teasdale, Brian Wilson, Nicola Tennant, Harry Burns, Alistair Darling and David Hamilton*

Glasgow, March 2016

Acknowledgements

We are very grateful to all the authors. The enthusiasm with which they accepted our invitations to contribute was clear and translated into willing responsiveness to meet editorial instructions and timelines. Their contributions produce the vivid portrayal of Sam that we hoped for.

The work of co-ordinating more than two dozen writers and editors was enormous and we are very grateful to Mrs Hilda Butler, Sam's constituency office secretary, for meeting this formidable challenge with such ability and dedication and so tactfully that everyone remained 'onside'.

We are grateful to Mrs Margaret Naismith for her skill in the assembly of all the material provided to our publisher.

We thank Birlinn for agreeing to publish our work and in particular we are grateful to Mr Tom Johnstone for support and guidance during its preparation and production.

The Royal College of Physicians and Surgeons of Glasgow and the University of Glasgow provided valuable practical support.

For permission to reproduce previously published material we thank the *Herald* (back cover photograph and 'Talking to Patients – The Golden Rules', page 198), the *Daily Record* (illustrations 7 and 10 in the plate section), the Press Association (front cover photograph), the *Scotsman* ('The Art of Moving Mountains', page 202) and the *West Highland Free Press* ('William Hutchison Murray: Larger-than-Life Hero of the Mountains', page 207).

Foreword

It is a pleasure to be part of this celebration of the life of Sam Galbraith. The turnout at his memorial service in the Bute Hall in the University of Glasgow on 26 August 2014 showed just how much he was admired, respected and loved by a wide range of people representing many different interests. His life and his career are covered in detail in the chapters that follow and this foreword sets the personal tone that runs through them.

Sam was a most distinguished graduate of the University of Glasgow. He was awarded a 1st class honours BSc in Anatomy in 1968 and graduated MB ChB with honours in 1971. His graduation brought him a number of prizes and in particular the Brunton Memorial Prize for the most distinguished graduate of the year. He completed this academic *tour de force* with an MD in 1976 on the subject of 'Acute traumatic intracranial haematoma'.

I met him as a student, but we really got to know each other when he became Hall Fellow in Surgery in 1973, a highly prestigious post. This was in the Department of Surgery in the Western Infirmary led by Sir Andrew Watt Kay. I had been Hall Fellow in the same Department four years before and was at that time a lecturer there. My annual salary as Hall Fellow was £1,400, so neither I nor Sam entered medicine for the money!

My colleagues from different parts of the medical world, including the British Medical Association, have been in touch with me to say how much they valued his clinical opinions, his skills as a surgeon, and his honesty and openness as Health Minister. They counted him as a friend. He was one of the few people who had an outstanding clinical career and subsequently moved into full-time politics.

Remembering Sam

His own clinical story is also enlightening. Lung fibrosis and a lung transplant provided for him real experience of the National Health Service and how valuable it was to everyone. This came through in his political career. His family, whom he loved dearly, were involved in this, as they were in all his initiatives, and they have our lasting gratitude for being with him through difficult times.

Sam and I met regularly across the years and always exchanged free and frank opinions! Every time we met he greeted me in the same way: 'Is that Wee Kenny?' he would say, usually out loud to the whole room. No matter how famous I became, what positions I held, and how tall I thought I was, it was always 'Wee Kenny'. That, I think, is why we got on so well and liked each other so much, together with his great courage.

It was a joy and a pleasure to have known Sam, and to watch his career grow and develop. I, like many others, miss him but we are grateful for the time we knew him and spent with him.

The story of Sam's life is as remarkable as it is varied. I hope you enjoy reading about his wide range of interests and his courage and remember him with affection and admiration.

Professor Sir Kenneth Calman KCB

Lecturer in Surgery 1970–74; Chief Medical Officer for Scotland, 1989–91, for England and Wales, 1991–97; Chancellor of the University of Glasgow, 2006 continuing.

Samuel Laird Galbraith: Chronology

18 October 1945–18 August 2014

Born	Clitheroe, Lancashire
Education	
1958–64	Greenock High School
1964–71	University of Glasgow

Degrees

1968	Bachelor of Science (BSc) with Honours 1st Class in Anatomy
1971	Medicinae Baccalaureus, Chirurgiae Baccalaureus (MB ChB) with Honours – Brunton Memorial Prize for most distinguished graduate in Medicine; Fullerton Prize; West of Scotland RAMC Memorial Prize
1975	Fellowship of Royal College of Physicians and Surgeons of Glasgow (FRCS Glasgow)
1977	Medicinae Doctor (MD), Glasgow
2002	Doctor of the University of Glasgow (DUniv) (Honorary)

Medical Appointments

1971–72	Pre-registration Junior House Officer, Western Infirmary, Glasgow
1972–79	Training in Surgery and Neurosurgery, Glasgow and Edinburgh

1976–77	MRC (Medical Research Council) Travelling Research Fellow, Department of Neurosurgery and Department of Neuroanatomy, Marine Bio-medical Institute, University of Texas, Galveston, Texas, USA
1979–88	Consultant Neurosurgeon, Institute of Neurological Sciences, Glasgow
1992	Honorary Senior Research Fellow, University of Glasgow

Visiting Neurosurgeon

1981	University of Zimbabwe
1985	Dartmouth College, Hanover, New Hampshire, USA
1994	Armed Forces Hospital, Dhahran, Saudi Arabia
1995	University of Hong Kong

Positions in Politics

1987–2001	Labour Member of Parliament for Strathkelvin and Bearsden
1988–92	Labour Shadow Health Spokesman
1992–93	Labour Shadow Employment Spokesman
1997–99	Parliamentary Under-Secretary of State for Scotland, Minister for Health and the Arts, Scottish Office, UK Government
1999–2001	Labour Member of Scottish Parliament for Strathkelvin and Bearsden
1999–2000	Minister for Children and Education (and the Arts), Scottish Executive
2000–01	Minister for Environment, Sport and the Arts, Scottish Executive

Other Appointments

1985–90	Elected Member, General Medical Council
1985–89	Chairman, Scottish Medical Aid for Nicaragua
1986–88	President, Medical Practitioners' Union
1986–88	Member of ASTMS National Executive Committee
1987–88	Chairman, Parliamentary Labour Party Devolution Committee – November 1987 assigned to draft Devolution Bill
2005–14	Specialist Medical Member, Tribunals Service, Scotland (Social Entitlement Chamber)
2006–14	Chair, Scottish Maritime Museum Trust
2006–14	General Medical Council (Fitness to Practise Panel)

Award

2016	Medal of the Society of British Neurological Surgeons

I

'The Child Is Father of the Man'

William Wordsworth, 1802, quoted in the Beach
Boys' song 'Surf's Up', 1971

Roderick, Nairn and Ailsa Galbraith

It is a salutary experience for the remaining siblings of a family of
five to reflect on the remarkable life of their late brother, Samuel
Laird Galbraith (Sam), who was the second child of their late
parents. The first was their late sister Katherine.

It is difficult to be precise about the sequence of events that
led to Sam's outstanding and varied career and his subsequent
health history. We begin here with memories of his childhood
and then youth, with Roderick, Nairn and Ailsa documenting
their family memories of Sam while leaving the details of the
other aspects of his life to close friends.

Sam was born on 18 October 1945 in a terraced house at 17
Nelson Street in the mill village of Low Moor, on the outskirts
of Clitheroe, Lancashire, into the loving care of devout Christian parents, Sam and Cathy Galbraith from Greenock. He,
like Roderick, was born there because Dad, on call-up for war
service, was posted to a training camp for engineers in the old
mill in the village.

Sam's father was a joiner and involved in the building of
Hatston Aerodrome in Orkney. Mother, who was a leading
Wren from Greenock and a member of the same church as our
father, was posted to Scapa Flow. They were married in Kirkwall
and spent a three-day honeymoon in a tent at Inganess Bay.

On being demobbed, Dad's CO called him in and, impressed by his instructor skills, recommended that he consider a teaching career and gave him an application form for teacher training. Dad entered Jordanhill College, in Glasgow, was first of his year in technical studies, took up a post at Greenock High School and was a technical teacher there for the rest of his career.

On the family's return to Greenock, accommodation was limited because of bomb damage and, being considered as incomers, they were at the bottom of the housing list. They moved into a bothy belonging to their friends, the Turners, at Branchton Farm. From there they moved to a tenement flat at (by an extraordinary coincidence) 17 Nelson Street, Greenock. This had a residency condition regarding the number of children the tenants could have. The figure was three and our mother was pregnant with Nairn, the fourth child.

With an eviction looming which would have split the family, and only limited help from the Council, Dad managed to secure a sublet flat at 49 Lynedoch Street. It was here that Roderick had his first coherent memories of stable family life.

The flat was on the third floor and contained a living room/kitchen with an old black range for heating, a 'set-in' double bed, a sink by the window and a gas cooker and two bedrooms. The stairwell was illuminated at night by gaslight, and down one flight of stairs was the toilet, shared by three families. Though it was basic and crowded by any of today's standards, our parents were just pleased to have a roof over their heads.

Despite hardships, this was a settled, happy time for the children and in June 1950 Nairn was born; this forename was our mother's maiden name.

The family environment was devoutly Christian and, although Sam would become an atheist in later life, it was from this upbringing, guided largely by our father, that Sam began to develop the values and principles that were to guide him in his sojourn through life.

The family routine was quickly established, and every Sunday we would be dressed for Sunday school, morning and afternoon. The appropriate dress included kilts, white shirts, jackets and Brylcreem on our hair. Here, even at this early age, Sam excelled in the Bible exams of the church, winning numerous prizes. On a few nice summer Sundays, our father would deviate from the normal route to the church and take a diversion through Lamont's ship repair yard next to the Custom House. There was no Health and Safety in those days, so Sam and Roderick, guided by Dad, could walk freely around the dry dock and watch the various workers engaged in the maintenance of the ships. For us all, this was fascinating and a delight, for it meant there would be no Sunday school that morning. The yard was wonderful and produced a resounding cacophony of noise and activity, but it was oh so antiquated. By the time we had finished, our father would say: 'Now, boys, don't tell your Mum that we didn't go to church.' These visits to the shipyards and docks had a lasting effect on the young Sam, and in later years he would recall the harsh, unhealthy and dangerous conditions he observed so early in his life.

Even in those days Lynedoch Street was busy with traffic, and in particular horses and carts transporting bags of raw sugar to the Westburn Refinery at the top end of the street. To refresh the horses there were water troughs at suitable intervals on the street, and on hot summer days, Sam and Roderick would fill these and then empty them into the gutter where they would float lollipop sticks, pretending they were boats in the ocean rapids.

During the summer, and on good days, Sam would lead the boys in search of adventure and walk up to the top of the street under the railway line to the perimeter of the Whinhill Golf Course marked by a dry-stone dyke. The boys called it 'The back of the wall'. It was a small raised area of grass in an otherwise soggy scrubland. Facing south it had the obvious advantage of the sun, together with a small stream gurgling close by. This Sam and Roderick would dam and then bathe in the peaty-coloured water; watercress grew just upstream and it was free.

Other days were spent fishing for the evening meal. This required digging ragworms at the start of the Esplanade for bait and then walking to the Custom House Quay to fish for cod and anything else that could be caught. On the dreich days when indoor confinement was accepted, the boys sometimes fished, in a competition, for socks on the kitchen floor by flinging hooks of open safety pins on lengths of wool from the set-in bed.

Sam, like most boys of his age, was also interested in football and, when not organising adventures or trips, could be found playing football on the back green of the tenement block across the street. These early games were perhaps the foundation of an interest in football that would remain with Sam for the rest of his life.

Sam had by now entered Mearns Street Primary School to which he and Katherine walked every day, about a half mile. Roderick recalls watching Sam sitting in front of the kitchen sink at a small table and practising 'joined-up writing'. He worked very hard at school, which became a characteristic of his life. His school report cards were full of excellent comments. In him there was a drive and a superior intellect that, in the years that followed, would set him apart from the crowd.

In those days holidays were in short supply, but when we did go, it was initially to Rose Cottage above Kames on the Kyles of Bute. It was delightfully quaint but had no running water or electricity. As for the toilet, Roderick says that he has no recollection of one. There was a well about 50 yards down a dirt track and a trickle of a burn to the side. Always seeking some adventure, the boys dammed this trickle to a depth of about two inches, whereupon Nairn, aged two, duly fell in head first and remained there. Roderick ran for help but Sam simply pulled him out.

For a reason that Roderick cannot remember, we had to visit the local doctor, and on the way back to the cottage Sam, aged six, announced that he was going to be a doctor. Our parents said something like: 'That's nice.' Little did we anticipate Sam's absolute focus on his dream future.

While at Kames we would fish for our tea, collect sea-coal from the shore (the coal was simply the spillage from the puffers unloading it onto the pier) and picnic at Ostel Bay or at the then tranquil remote inlet of Portavadie.

Exceptionally, at the age of six, Sam joined the Cub group of the West Kirk's Scouts (the Dandy 5th). Once again he excelled in a different competitive environment and enjoyed every minute of what he learnt there, tying knots, reading *The Jungle Book* and more. He rapidly became a Sixer and then the Senior Sixer. With the attainment of his Leaping Wolf, he went up to the Scout Troop. From Lynedoch Street to the Scout Hall was about two miles which he walked alone.

In 1954 the rules for house allocation in Greenock changed, and our family went to the top of the priority list. Accordingly we were offered and accepted a new three-bedroom semi-detached house, at 108 Braeside Road, on the very outskirts of the town in a partially completed council housing estate. Of cavity-wall construction, it consisted of a hall, living-room with fire, kitchen, dining-room, three bedrooms and, most importantly, a bathroom upstairs. A back boiler in the fire provided hot water and fed a partial central heating system. On the first night of occupancy, our mother kept the bedroom and bathroom doors open so that she could look into her first unshared toilet and bathroom. It was to us all paradise, and Friday night baths in the galvanised tub in front of the black range fire became a thing of the past!

The move to Braeside necessitated a move of schools, and Sam and Katherine, who were in the later stage of primary education, went to the Lady Alice Primary School, while Roderick went to Ravenscraig Primary School. Sam excelled, won several year prizes and in his final year was awarded Dux of the school.

At the end of the school year in 1955, the country experienced a prolonged summer heatwave. Every day during the holidays, except Sunday, Sam, Roderick and Jimmy McKirdy would walk along the old single-lane road towards Inverkip, past the head of the 'First Glen'. Here there had been an old millpond and several remains of the old mill in the glen were still just visible. From here the road passed Flaterton Farm, now worked by one of the Turner sons from Branchton Farm, and on towards the Second Glen. Just a few yards before the Glen, where there was a large wild cherry tree with bark to polish, we turned right through a gate into a field, over a stile and crossed the burn at the head of the glen. Then we went up a steep path crossing a pasture field to the final gate that opened up on to rough moorland. From there we followed the path between the hills to the left and the burn to the right until we passed through a dry-stone dyke towards a disused curling pond. After climbing over another stile into a fir-wood, we would drag an old thinned-out small tree down along a farm track, along a path down the side of a burn and across the main Greenock to Inverkip shore road. Crossing this, the path led to Lunderston Bay a few hundred yards ahead. There we lit a fire and boiled water from a nearby stream, and made soup from a packet. We had also brought with us a pot of stew, comprising link sausages, round sliced sausage, potatoes, onion, carrot and turnip, all provided by our mother. We played, explored, tried to swim and searched the rock pools. At 4.30 p.m., the mail boat, the *Saint Columba*, sailed by and it was time to head for home.

We mention all of the above, since Sam, at the age of nine, was responsible for us all and had to rein in Roderick's adventurous antics. Today, sixty years later, it is difficult to believe that any parent would allow their children such absolute freedom. These, however, were lonely places infrequently visited, and cars were rare. Nonetheless, for Sam this was the start of an incredibly formative time. He had the responsibility, made all the serious decisions and looked after us. What an upbringing of freedom, responsibility and care.

It was during August of 1955 that Ailsa was born, the final member of the Galbraith family. By all accounts, Sam at the age of ten (almost), and perhaps recognising the increased workload of our mother, regularly prepared the feed bottles for the new baby – a skill that Sam would perhaps put to good use in later life.

During the winter the boys were given hessian potato sacks from Davy Turner of Flaterton Farm and used them to stitch together a tent that they used in the garden and at Lunderston Bay. They even got a mention in the local newspaper. When it rained it simply poured in through the hessian. That year our parents bought a tent from the post office at the cost of £2.10s, a substantial cost for that day. It was made from offcuts of material. The tent was used for the first time at what we called the campsite, and the morning rain created a fine smirr of mist in the tent. For that first camp we had to make two transfers of kit from our house to the campsite. In the small tent were Sam, Roderick, Nairn, and our Dad. How small were we?

In the morning we got up. We had breakfast, played mock Highland games, then ate our lunch and waited for the farm cows to be taken for milking, when it would be time to go home. Unfortunately they were never taken in that day, and without a watch between us we simply decided to go home when we felt it was time; it happened to be only 12.30 in the afternoon. Our mother, who was 'sorting the house out', was not amused.

From our house at Braeside we were able to view the Renfrewshire Heights and in particular, a local knoll we called 'Sugar

Loaf Mountain' because of its profile, in front of Dunrod Hill. In that year, Dad, Sam, Roderick and Nairn left the house on an expedition to climb the said hill. Down the field we went to the Inverkip Road and across to the bridge over the River Kip and up to the railway crossing. From there it was a steep climb up Spango Glen to the Greenock Cut and onward past a bomb-crater to the summit. There we waved a white towel for our mother to see, but received no acknowledgement. She was busy elsewhere in the kitchen.

We then walked down to the Cut and on to the Glen Road. From there, without any map or local knowledge, we descended a most steep glen side to the water's edge. There we encountered a deep pool with a single large flat stone in the middle. It was surrounded by exquisite vegetation, undisturbed for generations. Young and old trees of birch, ash and others, enveloped the scene. Beautiful and enchanting as the scene was, its deeply shaded location did not entice us to stay, and so we pressed on up the glen.

On the west side and up a short slope, we encountered a flat soggy trail (later we would recognise it as the old rail track for the quarry).

As we ambled along the trail it suddenly opened up into a majestic clearing with a tall mature pine tree at the far right-hand side. Then to the left a fine natural swimming pool lay about 20 feet below in the curve of the glen. The excitement was palpable as we looked down on what was to become the scene of many swimming adventures. We called the clearing 'Lone Pine', and its loneliness remains to this day, albeit we spent many, many days there.

Lone Pine was not the best campsite, but further along and round an overgrown bend in the track was 'Apache Clearing', a flat sun-trap with sheep-cut grass, but unfortunately no swimming pool! Over time we dug a drainage ditch around the site and made it into a 'Robinson Crusoe Camp'.

A number of wooden planks discarded by the local farmer were put to good use, and we built a bridge across the Glen and made a diving-board from which we did deep dives into the pool and fished for minnows.

For an entire summer we ran barefoot through the glen and the bracken. Again, Sam was responsible for us all while we were free to indulge in our own adventurous activities. Each night we left the fire smouldering and covered with some turf. The next morning, on arrival, we blew on the embers and with some tinder brought the fire back into life.

Such was our attachment to 'Lone Pine' that we visited it every Boxing Day until both our father and Sam could no longer make it. In August 2015, Nairn, Ailsa and Roderick revisited 'Lone Pine' after many years' absence. The place was overgrown and the pool had to be viewed through the foliage. Without the sheep, nature returns.

The discovery of 'Lone Pine' had coincided with Sam joining the Scouts. Sam embraced the Scouts, and particularly the opportunity to camp every summer weekend at Everton Scout Camp above Inverkip. He progressed rapidly to become a Patrol Leader, Troop Leader and then an Officer (now called a Scout Leader). He also gained the highest award of becoming a Queen's Scout. He enjoyed being in charge and leading his patrol and the troop. Focused on the adventure side of scouting, Sam was always organising and leading activities such as winter work parties at Everton, weekend 'wild' camping and, of course, hill-walking. It was not unusual for Scouts to turn up at the Friday night meeting with full rucksacks and at 9 p.m. to leave on a midnight hike to Everton via the Cut and Daff Dam.

The Dandy 5th, at that time, was a remarkable troop. At one ceremony they had 11 Queen's Scouts presented with their certificates and regularly won all the competitions available: the Shannon Cup for Scouting, the Pioneering Trophy and the

County Flag. The majority of these exceptional Scouts, led by Sam, went on to have very successful professional careers.

One of the tasks during a Shannon Cup Competition was to make tea in a paper bag. The accepted method is to hold the empty bag over the hot embers of a spent fire to warm it. Thereafter cold water is dripped in over some tea-leaves, while the bottom of the bag is kept dry by the heat of the embers. All the troops but the 5th presented the examiners with a pile of wet mush. To the examiners' amazement, the 5th successfully made proper tea in a paper bag. Their success was due to Sam spotting the ambiguity in the statement of the task, that is: 'To make tea in a paper bag'. Accordingly we heated the bag over hot embers, dropped in some tea-leaves and then carefully dripped in boiling water. This was not cheating, for do you boil the water in the teapot? Sam simply interpreted the loose wording of the task to our advantage.

Each examiner had breakfast made for him or her, and after having eaten they graded the efforts. Sam in his usual way started by making a practice version, which became the breakfast of one of the patrol members. The next attempt was better and so on, until the bacon, eggs and beans were spot on and served up to the examiners. As for the other troops, they produced the usual messed-up food.

Sam arranged a midweek working party prior to the competition where we would search for dry, dead firewood, chop it up and hide it in preparation for the competition. There was also a back-up couple of Scouts hiding in the woods to provide help, if needed. The Scout motto is: 'Be prepared'.

One of the tasks in the pioneering competition was to build a Roman catapult. These were substantial structures, some 12-feet high with an A-frame at each end. The objective was to hit a target or throw a projectile as far as possible. At the end of the day the trials began, and our construction was positively dire. The projectile hardly cleared the catapult, and so the other troops went to bed in a very happy and contented state. After all, had they not got the better of the 5th at last? Our secret weapons, Sam and Roderick, then came into play. They both discussed the problem, and having worked out the solution, went into the woods to secure a long-dead and dry fir tree that was slender at the top and thick at the bottom. They also found a strong, stopper log that would instantaneously arrest the catapult's rotation prior to the vertical. This they positioned and adjusted until the optimum stopping point was located. It was a rare occasion when Sam, the leader of the patrol, accepted Roderick's analysis and choice of timber. When the morning came we were ready, and to the utter surprise of the other troops who had seen our pathetic efforts the day before, we were busy and confident. When we pulled the trigger rope the slender tree bent and stored up potential energy. When the thick end of the tree hit the stopper log ahead of the vertical, it released its stored energy in a whiplash and threw the projectile way beyond the target distance. On the second, less violent attempt we hit the target. No other troop managed to get near to the target and the 5th won the trophy.

While an officer, Sam realised that his interests were changing; his friends had all left the troop and the call of the mountains beckoned, particularly in the winter. Like everything else in life, the Scouts had had their day.

When Sam entered secondary school, a prerequisite for going on to study medicine was Latin. A Dux of his primary school, he was automatically selected by the Latin principal. His Latin exam marks were outstanding with an average of about 95 per cent. A year later, the requirement for medical students to have Latin was dropped, and his marks plummeted to lower than 10 per cent. If you don't need it, don't suffer it was Sam's attitude. Sam worked hard in senior school balancing his studies with other interests and gained all the necessary subjects, qualifications and grades to be offered a place at Glasgow University Medical School.

His enthusiasm for football saw him successfully trial and play right-back (there were different positions in those days) for the school from first to third year. The interest continued throughout his life as a spectator, first with Greenock Morton and then with Rangers. In later years, when studying, he would come down from his room to watch *Scotsport* on TV with Arthur Montford. More recently, at a family gathering, Sam disappeared after dinner to be found in the study watching a football match!

He joined the school rowing club that was organised by the Deputy Rector in his fourth year. The training was mainly in sea boats or racing shells, and he rowed for the school at bow in a four and a shared eight with the Royal West of Scotland Amateur Boat Club. In his sixth year, having already gained a place at medical school, he spent most of his time at the Boat Club.

Also in his fourth year, he joined the school debating society (the Forum), again run by the Deputy Rector, and by all accounts Sam was a robust debater. Perhaps an indication of what was to come.

It was probably Sam who made the preliminary diagnosis of the most debilitating malady that Roderick encountered in his life. In Sam's third year at University, one Friday night in late January 1966, Roderick took ill while with a friend in Inverkip. He was in severe pain and a doctor was called. He was a little upset at being called out but administered pain relief; it didn't work. From somewhere our father enlisted the help of a friend with a car and got Roderick back to Braeside. He was in a dreadful state, and his own doctor diagnosed a 'blinding migraine'. All night Sam lay awake listening to the sounds of Roderick's agony, and in the morning he took charge and told our father to get a second opinion. The doctor duly arrived; he spoke with

Sam and then went upstairs to where Roderick lay. No examination was necessary as one look was enough for him to order Roderick's transfer to a local hospital. It was Sam who realised that the two previous doctors hadn't taken in the full seriousness of the haemorrhage Roderick had suffered. It was his initiative that set the further investigation and treatment in motion.

During this very trying time for the family, one evening, while at home waiting for news from our parents at Killearn Hospital, Sam commented to Nairn that if Roderick pulled through, he would specialise in neurosurgery. It was not until Sam himself was in a precarious state after his lung transplant that he told Roderick he was the reason he became a neurosurgeon. Well, after surgery and much time, Roderick recovered and carried on with life, gaining a PhD in aerodynamics and pursuing a successful career in academia.

For Sam, his childhood days were over and he had taken a major step on the path to the career he had chosen, all those years ago at the age of six.

Roderick Galbraith

The Shoda Professor of Aerospace Engineering, University of Glasgow, retired 2011.

Nairn Galbraith

Manager, Hebrides Missile Range, retired 2007.

Ailsa Galbraith

Physics Teacher, Park Mains School, Erskine, retired 2014.

2

Fort William, Study and Survival

Ewan Macdonald

Sam was accepted for medicine and started the University of Glasgow course in 1964, when he took the first three years of an MB ChB. He then changed to a BSc in pure science, and was awarded a BSc with 1st class honours in anatomy in November 1968.

He completed the MB ChB course, and graduated on 9 July 1971, winning the top prize, the Brunton Memorial Prize, the West of Scotland RAMC Memorial Prize (Royal Army Medical Corps) and the Fullerton Prize.

His entry into the University was relatively unremarkable and he joined the rowing club and the Labour Party. He was initially inhibited from full participation socially by being one of the many Glasgow students who lived at home, which was then a West of Scotland tradition for economic reasons.

He had had a dalliance with the Communist Party prior to coming to the University, and his strong socialist principles were evident from the beginning. He liked to suggest that he came from a rather more disadvantaged family and community than was the case: his dad, a quiet, strong and lovely man was a secondary school teacher, while his mother was an equally kind person and the rock of the large and successful family.

As he settled into academic life Sam's personality soon emerged. In those days there was a higher proportion of privately educated students in the medical year, whom Sam regarded as some kind of alien species and loved to bait.

He was outspoken, and often scathing and humorously satirical. However, there was something unique about him from the outset which I still find hard to define. His eyes were always engaging and direct, his smile had a mischievous wickedness, and the tone of his voice was such that, whatever insult he pronounced in his broad West of Scotland tones as he portrayed himself as 'one of the workers', his underlying character and endearing qualities communicated themselves subliminally to all. It was generally thought that he could 'get away with murder' with what he said, and he did!

Initially his political incorrectness knew no bounds, as he expounded about women, marriage, public-school boys and girls, social elites, the privileged, right-wing politicians, and the churches in general. Whether he would have been accepted for medical school today is questionable, as he certainly would not fit into the highly coached psychometrically tested cohort of worthy individuals that we now see. Today no 'characters' are allowed and he certainly was one.

But, on reflection, he was so intelligent and intuitive that he probably would have been able to present himself in his interviews and written statement in such a way as to meet all the appropriate selection standards. Despite his initial outspoken critiques of all, with advancing maturity he became one of the most tolerant of individuals, but could still be wicked in debate!

For some of us going to university, staying in a hall of residence meant access to continuous dissolute ribaldry, communal celebration of everyone's birthday at the Three in One or the Halt bars, followed by all-night parties or bridge games to the sound of Manfred Mann, and the inevitable resits of exams. In our hall of residence there was one exception, a fellow medical student who did nothing but study and who wondered, of Sam: 'Who is this guy who got results as good or better than me when I studied all the time?'

Sam, when he was not living at home, was such a live-wire that it seemed that his brilliance was effortless and it was only in researching this chapter that I learned that he shared a bedroom with Roderick and Nairn, and Roderick recounts that he 'worked all the time, and all night'. He had once asked Sam, on seeing a well-thumbed copy of the massive *Gray's Anatomy*, if he had actually read it?

'Yes, several times,' was the response.

Sam invited him to open it and suggested that Roderick read any sentence. When Roderick obliged, Sam continued the paragraph from memory.

Roderick, thinking this was a chance event, turned to another section and read a sentence, and again Sam continued the paragraph from memory.

As Sam progressed through the course his personality developed, and in lectures he could combine rapt attention with wicked humour, being brilliant at the *sotto voce*, calling out from the back of the lecture hall when the diminutive Professor of Anatomy, G.M. Wyburn, was lecturing: 'Get aff yer knees!' As usual, this did not destroy his career and he progressed to an intercalated BSc in Anatomy, achieving 1st class honours. A robust female medical student, who was a year behind him on the same course towards an Honours BSc, reports that she found him 'terrifying' because of his intellectual dominance and his humour.

He was the master of the one-line put-down; and a tall, suave contemporary, later a distinguished President of a Royal College, who was on very good terms with Sam, recalls getting into a crowded hospital lift which was filled with visitors and other staff. After an amiable exchange of greetings, Sam suddenly announced: 'I am much more cultured than you, you bastard!' to which there could be no response! As ever, Sam got away with this and was never the subject of a complaint to the GMC or anyone else.

Another contemporary observes that he was like Socrates, and could interject a comment into the conversation which would subsequently lead to furious debate.

His propensity later for practical joking has been reliably reported. Once when Sam was on duty in the Western Infirmary, he surreptitiously fed a hose-pipe from the room above down and through the window and into the bed of his colleague on duty, perfectly timing the turning on of the tap after the latter had retired for well-needed sleep with a lady companion.

The Belford Years

The Belford Hospital in Fort William has for long welcomed medical student placements and has a long history of providing a great clinical apprenticeship for medical students and producing distinguished doctors. Around his fourth year, while doing his BSc, Sam appeared at the Belford where I, as a local, had spent much time, and there our friendship developed. The Belford dealt and deals with much acute illness, mountain-rescue casualties and road accidents, and has a surgical unit, a smaller medical unit and an obstetric unit, then GP- and now midwife-led. All was then under the amiable supervision of the solitary consultant surgeon, the legendary Iain Campbell; Edinburgh-trained (white coat-collar always up), of great presence, but despite that of Argyllshire origin and with an enormous affinity for the Highlander. There, for the first and only time I was able to teach Sam, showing him how to clerk in a patient.

Sam was staying in the hospital and became very popular with the all the patients, staff, cleaners, cooks and reception staff, and became the unofficial social convener for the younger unattached nurses. We got experience of stitching, taking bloods, assisting in theatre, attending clinics and seeing casualties. Sam's personality quickly impressed everyone, and he was a frequent visitor to my family home, where he initially appalled my father with his eating habits, which were another anti-establishment demonstration of bad behaviour. However my parents were very fond of him, and when he arrived somehow the room lit up, and that was a characteristic throughout his life.

At that time, like many medical students, he fluctuated between serial binge-drinking and extreme abstinence, arriving one New Year at my home and refusing all drams. However his abstinence did not get in the way of patient care, and he went round the wards after that midnight to give all the *cailleachs* (old women) and *bodachs* (old men) who were fit enough, a wee whisky or sherry. In these days alcohol could be prescribed.

It was in Fort William that our mutual interest in climbing developed, Sam having been introduced to it by Roderick on a visit when they went to the Poll Dubh Slabs in Glen Nevis. Roderick recounts that from the outset it was obvious that Sam was a much better climber than he was.

Sam and I would escape to local crags at every opportunity and my memory is of terrific evenings in the sunshine, with only a few midges, testing ourselves out on ever harder routes and always arguing about something.

We graduated to snow and ice climbing and decided to do the easiest gully on Ben Nevis – Red Gully – and Sam invited a gentle, shy Indian doctor trainee to come, advising him to be warmly dressed. Our colleague duly presented himself in his suit, shirt and tie, and a long black woollen overcoat, wearing normal shoes, and so off we went. Sam had an old wooden-shafted long Alpenstock which he gave me, while he used something slightly more modern. He always had better gear than me, and seemed to have more money despite the professed hardship of his upbringing, because he was always winning bursaries and class prizes.

We proceeded up the exciting Gully. We had an old hemp rope of dubious condition and securely tied our Indian colleague in the middle. Sam led and soon we all emerged at the top into a glorious warm sunset, elated with the experience.

Enthused by our prowess, Sam suggested that the two of us do a much more serious proposition – Gardyloo Gully. So, as very early customers of Nevisport, we bought crampons and some slings and a 'deadman', i.e. a snow anchor. Ice daggers were then in vogue (they were useless) and I couldn't afford one, so borrowed one of my mother's large kitchen knives.

Dressed in woolly jumpers and tweed breeches, Sam with his old Harris tweed jacket and cagoule and me with a black plastic fishing jacket, we set off on the long walk in and then up the progressively steepening Observatory Gully toward the Gardyloo Gully at the very top. We learned a valuable lesson by stopping too late to put on our crampons on a very steep, icy 2,000-foot slope, before we reached the snow cave at the bottom of a vertical ice chimney and wall. By this time it was cold, windy and spindrift was coming down and it was all feeling very serious. I buried the deadman anchor in the snow and the bold Sam led off up the vertical iced chimney with the old 80-foot grey hemp rope attached. He was soon out of sight and earshot, and the rope went tight and was being tugged. I realised he had probably not reached the top and set off quickly, dragging the deadman behind with the fairly useless alpenstock ice axe in one hand and Mum's kitchen knife in the other. I had to traverse out of the chimney onto a vertical face of ice; the specially sharpened kitchen knife couldn't penetrate the hard ice, so I had to put it between my teeth. Fortunately previous climbers had cut steps and there were good ice handholds; up I went into the spindrift hoping that Sam, at least, was secure. The rope stayed tight and eventually we made it, emerging on the summit plateau to be greeted by the astonished looks of walkers on the summit. Survival gave us a feeling of ecstasy, and it was during that later profound philosophical analysis which can only occur in the moderately inebriated we came to the conclusion that the experience was more exciting than sex.

Sam's subsequent mountain exploits are recorded elsewhere, but some extended into more local activity, such as when he decided to climb the Brodick Church steeple one evening, falling after about 15 feet into the caring hands of the local police!

There are several – possibly apocryphal – accounts of Sam being invited to police stations because of overly social activities. Both as a student and later in his career, his favourite response to the question about his occupation was: 'I'm a brain surgeon.' To which the response was usually: 'Aye, right, I heard that one before.' When outdoors, his general air of scruffiness and effervescence always led to scepticism about his day job. On one occasion the police phoned Professor Bryan Jennett to ask if it was indeed the case that he was a surgeon, which led to the usual admonition and release.

He continued to be politically active, and a friend recalls entering the University Union where Sam was selling a far-left newspaper. He asked Sam what he was doing that for and got the usual response about supporting the workers. 'But Sam, selling newspapers is really a waste of your time.' At which, after momentary reflection, Sam responded: 'Yes, you are quite right.' When discussing Sam's student years everyone laughs and offers another anecdote.

It is quite impossible for me to think of Sam without smiling. He was a much-loved character who was humorous, abrasive, infuriating and challenging, but always popular with all, both with his patients and the pompous alike, and always radiating compassion for the disadvantaged.

Ewan Macdonald

Medical Student, University of Glasgow 1964–70; Professor, Health Working Lives Group, University of Glasgow, 1990–2016.

3

Camaraderie Was the Order of the Day

Bill Murray

Sam Galbraith and I began medical school in Glasgow together in 1964. On the way through we each gained an additional intercalated science degree (BSc honours) before graduating as doctors seven years later. By that time Sam's range of unique qualities was becoming evident. His final year book quotes of 'Rubbish! *ipse dixit ad nauseam*' and 'I have an inferiority complex – everyone's inferior to me', while characteristically (probably) tongue in cheek, were preludes to qualification with honours and the class prize.

We then spent the next twelve months as junior house officers (JHOs) in general surgery and general medicine as required by the GMC for full registration. Sam and I were resident JHOs in Professor Andrew Kay's surgical unit in the Western Infirmary, Glasgow. Residents were aptly named: we had a bedroom in the hospital, a residents' mess, ate in the staff canteen and were provided with supper in the evenings. For an average of one hundred and thirty hours per week we received £980 per year before tax. Camaraderie and mutual support were the rule amongst residents.

Weekday responsibilities began at 7.30 a.m. and went on until the work was done. This included taking all the blood samples (to be done before the first ward round or there was trouble), attending all ward rounds and taking instructions, arranging investigations, prescribing drugs, writing progress notes, clerking in new admissions, carrying out practical procedures such as male catheterisation and setting up intravenous infusions, taking consent for surgery, preparing theatre lists for typing, retrieving and filing the results of investigations, writing immediate discharge letters and dealing with the day-to-day clinical problems that arise in every surgical ward.

There was a JHO for the male ward and one for its female counterpart. Out-of-hours cover was shared in a 1 in 2 rota. On duty during a weekday night, Sam would work until dinnertime in his own ward before covering both wards until the next morning. He then completed another day's work in his own ward before handing over cover to his colleague. He could then leave the hospital if he wished. Every second weekend a resident covered both wards from 6 p.m. on Friday until Monday morning before completing his own ward work for that day. Every fourth day was 'receiving': assessing and managing patients sent in by GPs or self-attending. Both residents usually worked until midnight on weekday receiving; at weekends one JHO dealt with all emergencies for 24 hours.

How did Sam cope with all this? The reader will not be surprised to learn that Sam thrived, quickly discovering the secrets of becoming a very good resident. He worked hard, learnt to distinguish between the important and the things that could be left on the back burner; he knew his patients in great detail and understood their management plans. Just after he started, he went to the X-ray booking office with a bottle of whisky and a large box of chocolates, introducing himself as Sam from Professor Kay's unit. The other surgical residents couldn't understand how Sam's patients always had their X-rays done so quickly!

Surgical residents were required to work for three weeks in the 'Casualty' Department which then consisted of two rooms in the bowels of the hospital, staffed by a surgical SHO (senior house officer), a surgical JHO and experienced nurses. The patients were defined by the porters as having a 'condition of " . . . "', Sam's favourite being 'condition of lower body'! Shortly after our time the hospital management decided it was wrong to have initial triage carried out by porters and replaced them with nurses. A survey after the change revealed that re-referral rates had been lower with porter triage!

When a resident was away from the ward, usually a final-year medical student stood in. Sam's co-resident went to Casualty over the festive season and a student locum was not available. Not a problem for Sam – he just looked after the whole of Professor Kay's unit for three weeks solid, only getting occasional cross-cover in the evenings. He managed to dress up as Santa Claus to distribute presents to the patients still in hospital on Christmas Day, and then confused several children when spotted later in Byres Road being assisted back from the Aragon pub with two other Santas and a fairy.

Sam enjoyed working in casualty: stitching lacerations, reading X-rays and treating simple fractures and sprains. One evening the waiting room was full and the nurses knew it would take a long time to clear the backlog. Sam put on his old coat and bunnet and shuffled into the waiting room. He stood for a time then announced in a strong Greenock accent: 'This is dreadful. Ah'm awa to the Royal, it's much faster there.' He walked out, followed by most of the mobile potential patients.

Sam found his time in general medicine less interesting than surgery. Things moved too slowly; there was too much discussion without action. He considered many tests ordered by his 'seniors' to be useless and unnecessary, and if asked, he would make up the result. He wasn't scared to debate patient investigation and management and the 'rubbish!' count was high during his medical residency.

Sam and I came together again in August 1973 when we commenced surgical training in the Western Infirmary; I joined

Professor Kay's unit as the senior house officer while Sam held the prestigious post of Hall Fellow, the gift of the Professor himself. We were each keen to experience and learn as much as possible, as quickly as possible, and used to commiserate with each other that we were simply being used as 'a pair of hands in theatre and a pair of feet on the ward round'. We were still on call every second night and every second weekend, but now didn't have to live in the hospital except on receiving days. Cameraderie was still high and practical jokes not uncommon. One of our residents regarded himself as a bit of a ladies' man and boasted that he planned to bring back a young lady to his room to show off his etchings! Sam used his climbing skills to get along the outside wall of the hospital, enter the resident's room on the second floor through the window and open the door from the inside. I had been informed that a large latex theatre glove could be expanded with water to reach the size of a small pig if this was carried out in a half-filled bath with a sheet under the glove to allow it to be gently transported thereafter. It worked; the glove was duly deposited on the resident's bed and covered with a blanket. There was no more boasting!

Sam and I thoroughly enjoyed our time in Professor Kay's surgical unit and worked well together. In December 1973 my wife had to undergo induction to deliver our first child, but on the appointed date I was first on call receiving and couldn't leave the hospital. When Sam found out what was happening he just said 'For ----'s sake, Bill, give me your pager and go away!' A few weeks later I was again receiving SHO when I got an urgent phone call from my wife. The solution this time was provided by 'wee Kenny' Calman (surgical registrar – now Sir Kenneth Calman) who walked up Byres Road and bought baby bottles and a steriliser for us.

Sam never tried to convert his junior medical colleagues to his political views, but as SHOs I did try to tease him about his car. He drove a very trendy MGB sports coupé, and I asked him how he could square this with his political stance. He replied quickly that, in his opinion, 'Everyone should have an MGB GT.' Sam clearly had great respect for his parents. When he went down to Greenock for a weekend home visit he always spent some time cleaning out the inside of his car to make sure that all the empty beer bottles and cans were removed.

We worked hard as JHOs and SHOs, spent a lot of our lives in the hospital and were part of a team providing outstanding continuity of patient care. As our seniors observed our progress we were given increasing responsibility, which encouraged our desire to develop further. However, the work of a surgical unit was very different then from now, and our wards contained many patients making an uncomplicated recovery from surgery and who needed not much more than nursing care. Today only sick patients remain in surgical wards, activity is intense and junior doctors work under extreme pressure. They have lost the experience of team-work and the continuity of patient care that Sam and I valued.

The BSc degrees that Sam and I gained had implanted an interest in the research which we knew was required to further our careers. In August 1973 Sam set up a prospective clinical study of the relationship between alcohol consumption and head injury and the effect of alcohol on the conscious level of injured patients. He asked me to help and we studied 918 consecutive patients with a head injury admitted to the Western Infirmary over the next year. Of these admissions, 47 per cent occurred on either a Friday or a Saturday night and 62 per cent had alcohol in their blood. The mean level of blood alcohol on any day was 193mg/100ml. The highest blood alcohol level recorded was 378mg/100ml – in a patient noted as being 'drowsy'! Depression of the conscious level began to occur at blood alcohol levels around 200mg/100ml, but a substantial number of patients in coma had a serious head injury. The study suggested that it would be dangerous to attribute reduced conscious level in a head injury patient to alcohol intoxication alone unless their blood alcohol level was well over 200mg/100ml. The catchment area of the Western Infirmary had certainly proved fruitful for the study in Glasgow. The work was presented at various meetings and published in 1976 and 1977 along with a book chapter in 1977. Sam's study was the start of his neurosurgical publications.

After Sam began neurosurgical training in 1974, at the Institute of Neurological Sciences at the Southern General Hospital, our careers and friendship continued in parallel. Sam was challenging and stimulating to be with. He didn't tolerate fools, bluffers or shirkers and could switch into misogynist mode to cause resentment. He was honest and forthright, often to the point of being rude if taken the wrong way. But he also was extremely intelligent and talented, great fun to be with, reliable, trustworthy, someone who would help if he possibly could. At the packed memorial event held in the Bute Hall of Glasgow University after Sam's death, I reflected on my belief that my 'rubbish!' count was low and that made me proud.

Bill Murray

Junior House Officer, Trainee, Senior Lecturer in Surgery, Western Infirmary, Glasgow, 1971–89; Consultant Surgeon, Royal Infirmary, Glasgow, 1989–2007.

4

An Extraordinary Neurosurgeon, Colleague and Friend

Graham Teasdale

In 1967, when I came from south of the border to Glasgow to teach anatomy, Sam Galbraith was already in the Department doing the research that led to his BSc with honours. Even as a third year medical student he was showing the incisive intellect that became his trademark; he had already authored a communication in the *Lancet* and clearly was outstanding academically.

He was hard-working but also played hard. The Department's social life centred around its football team in which Sam was a tough defender, in the mould of Billy Bremner and Dave Mackay of those times. I was drafted in for a vital match. Soon after the start of the game I set off after a ball sent up the wing, felt a sudden, sharp, severe pain in the back of my leg just above the ankle, and fell. Recognising a ruptured Achilles tendon, I said, 'I need an ambulance, I have to go hospital.' The comment came back – if I wasn't such a big English Jessie I could surely manage to stay and play on the wing, at least until half-time.

So began 47 years of firm friendship, over which I saw, and for several years shared, Sam's life as student, trainee doctor and consultant neurosurgeon, followed by his transition to politician and finally retirement.

When Sam finished his student career he already had a commitment to neurosurgery. This ambition had been implanted when his younger brother, Roderick, had an operation in the

Glasgow Unit for a brain haemorrhage. So, immediately after the usual pre-registration junior medical and surgical posts, he sought practical experience of neurosurgery in short posts in Glasgow and Edinburgh. In 1974, after two years in general surgery, he chose to begin training in the Glasgow Neurosurgical Unit, bringing us together again because I was then the senior registrar.

The Glasgow Unit was the ideal place for Sam. In 1970, for the first time outside London, neurosurgery had been brought together with its allied specialities of neurology, neuroradiology, neuropathology, neurophysiology and neuroanaesthesia in a new, purpose-built 'Institute of Neurological Sciences' (INS). This served all the three million people in the West of Scotland, was well resourced and in the vanguard of providing the latest technological advances. The Neurosurgical Unit had a longstanding ethos of team-working and recently had gained an extra, academic dimension through the creation of a University Department of Neurosurgery. This was led by Professor Bryan Jennett, the outstanding neurosurgical thinker of the time. Bryan was to be an inspiration and a career-long mentor to Sam and myself.

The exciting, heady environment created by this combination of a busy surgical service, driven by a scientific clinical culture, provided a foundation on which Sam flourished. Indeed, he burst on the neurosurgical scene.

During his early surgical posts Sam had become interested in head injuries – especially in the risk of the development of a blood clot on the brain. This was much feared by the general surgeons who then looked after most victims. Between 1973 and 1976 he published three landmark papers in the *Lancet* and the *British Medical Journal*. These analysed the early features in the cases of a large number of people in whom the complication had actually occurred. Sam's results showed that in almost all adults there were warning signs from the start. This meant that the prevalent policy of the time of admitting for observation thousands of head-injured people with a normal neurological state and negative skull X-ray was unnecessary, and, what's more, ineffective. These were damning faults to Sam's critical thinking. His findings pointed to how a more rational, risk-based approach using information on age, clinical findings and X-ray findings could be used to limit admission to those most likely to benefit.

Sam was awarded an MD for his work. It set the scene for risk-based guidelines for the use of CT scanning that came a few years later and that led to progressive improvements in outcome of people with a head injury. Rigorous thinking, careful investigation focused on something practically important that made things better for people – the characteristic Galbraith approach. Serious but never dull. He found that many head injuries followed alcohol consumption and added a new condition to the medical lexicon – the 'moving pavement syndrome'. An early example of his ability to find a memorable phrase.

Sam was then awarded a much sought-after travelling scholarship from the Medical Research Council. He spent this in Galveston in the United States, where he returned to the electron microscopy of his BSc and produced new, fundamental anatomical findings. When Sam left for America we weren't sure what he would make of Texans or what they would make of Sam. As Gary Wilhelm describes in his chapter, it proved interesting for both sides!

Sam passed swiftly through clinical training. He was described by Mr Alistair Paterson, the senior neurosurgeon and himself the doyen of his generation, as the most talented trainee there had been in Glasgow. This was an era that included future professors of neurosurgery in Edinburgh, London, Cambridge, Southampton, Newcastle and centres across the world. After he became a consultant in 1979 at the then unusually young age of

32, Sam and Alistair formed a happy, productive team and an enduring friendship.

As a surgeon, Sam was outstandingly skilful, with an economical, instinctive technique that made the difficult seem simple. The rest of us encouraged him to specialise in operations on an artery, the basilar, that lies in the very middle of the head under the base of the brain. Gaining access to repair the artery after it had bled was one of the most complex and demanding procedures. Determined to achieve excellence, Sam went to Canada to learn the latest microsurgical technique from Dr Charles Drake, then the world's leading expert. Later, when the patients Sam had treated were reviewed, their outcomes were equal to the best in the world.

In the late 1970s the customary approach to consultant practice was the traditional hierarchical model, with a surgeon exclusively responsible for 'his' (very occasionally 'her') patients. Discussion of the management of a patient of another surgeon was rare in most units but was the rule in Glasgow. This happened at twice weekly 'X-ray' conferences attended by all surgeons – consultants and juniors, radiologists and other specialists, the forerunner of today's 'Multi-Disciplinary Team' (MDT) meetings.

Debate was robust. Sam was usually provocative and forthright, especially if the meeting was dull or if there was a hint of loose thinking. 'What did you do that for?' would come the challenge. But he was equally open to questioning of his actions, and his views were never expressed with malice. Instead they were intended to provoke the vigorous, open discussion that often improved management and informed and opened the minds of trainees. This culture of self-scrutiny was a key characteristic of the Unit and we believed it provided the best safeguard for patients. Sam's experiences were no doubt reflected in his definition, when Minister for Health in 1998, of clinical governance as 'corporate accountability for clinical performance' – by far the most insightful and useful description of a much-touted concept.

In contrast to the scrutiny of unit meetings, consultants see little of each other's day-to-day relationships with patients, junior colleagues and other health care staff. But all knew that Sam the surgeon was also a doctor in the best sense. He treated people with empathy and as equals; he could raise serious topics but tinge their discussion with humour. He valued the contributions of everyone in the neurosurgical team. No matter your background, qualifications or status, if you were doing your best for people you had Sam's respect and backing. To trainees he was an excellent teacher, an ally in encouraging their development. When one registrar was asked what was his ambition the answer was simple: to become Mr Galbraith. With more senior colleagues, as well as being challenging, Sam knew when to be considerate and supportive – both professionally and personally – to myself and no doubt others at difficult times.

It is sometimes questioned if Sam might have followed a fully academic career, with a university department his natural home. But he seemed to value the independence an NHS post gave him, relishing the freedom to chart his own course without the responsibilities for organisation and fundraising that he would probably have found tedious. As it was, he showed how at that time a consultant in the NHS could combine a full load of clinical service with substantial research activity. He was effectively an extra member of the Glasgow University Department.

We worked together closely and productively on studies that increased understanding and improved practical management of patients with a head injury. Sam also published studies on several other topics, including boxing and fatalities from climbing, and helped Bryan Jennett to revise his popular textbook *An Introduction to Neurosurgery*. We presented papers at conferences in many parts of the world, promoted the use of the Glasgow Coma Scale and the profile of the Glasgow Unit.

Hospitality enjoyed abroad had to be returned. When the delegates to a conference in Glasgow found their enjoyment of a boat trip on Loch Katrine threatened by a downpour, Sam produced a crate of 'Scotland's national drink'. This rescued the occasion. It was acclaimed by all to be much superior to the Asian or American versions of the spirit and to local brews such as Maotai and sake that we had laboured so earnestly to become attuned to.

After almost a decade in neurosurgery, and despite or perhaps because of his success, it seemed that Sam was becoming restless. He needed a new challenge, an opportunity to change things on a much bigger scale than was possible through the medical profession alone. Also, I learnt later, he had become aware that he had developed a serious illness that meant that the time available to him to achieve change might be very short.

Sam had pulmonary fibrosis, a rare condition, then also known as fibrosing alveolitis. In this, scarring and hardening develop in the lungs, which lose their elasticity and are less able to take in air. The result is severe, progressively worsening and eventually constant shortness of breath, so that even speaking becomes impossible. The condition is poorly understood. In the 1980s, as now, there was no effective medical treatment and victims could expect to live for only a few years.

Sam's selection as a Labour Party candidate for Parliament in 1987 provided the opportunity to embark on initiating change. The remarkable lasting success of his lung transplant in 1990, which was then a rare, almost experimental procedure, allowed him to see many changes come to fruition.

Election came very much to Sam's surprise. His colleagues searched for a way that he could continue to combine the two activities, knowing he would give fully to both. But for an

MP, employment by the NHS was ruled out. Sam reluctantly resigned. This was a great loss to Glasgow, both for his skills and for his example of how neurosurgery should be practised.

Sam never lost an interest in neurosurgical matters, and for a few years, during parliamentary breaks, he was able to put his surgical skills to use in other parts of the world. A fellowship with the University enabled him to continue in research and might have provided a re-entry to neurosurgery as an alternative to a life on the back-benches. In the end politics prevailed.

Fortunately our contacts and friendship continued through our adjacent holiday homes on the shore of Loch Fyne. Over the years, we watched our families grow. Sam and his family and friends watched my early attempts to water ski with great mirth, but a few years later his girls, including Nicola, appreciated a tow behind my boat to 'get up' – which they did at the very first attempt.

An opportunity for amusement at Sam's expense came when he launched his new boat; as it pulled away from the beach, we on shore could see it was slowly sinking lower and lower in the water. Fortunately our shouts were heard and the boat was beached safely. Sam had forgotten to put the bung in! On another occasion the INS hill-walking group stayed at a remote Highland hotel where en-suite facilities were unknown. During the night Sam went to the bathroom, his room door closed and he had neither key nor pyjamas. A career in brain surgery does not guarantee practicality – but dealing with crises becomes second nature!

Increasingly, as time passed, we reminisced about how it had all been different in our day. And perhaps there was some truth in this. We counted ourselves as the lucky generation, because we had seen dramatic advances – operating using a microscope had made surgery precise and safe, CT and MRI scanning made it possible to see inside the head without drilling a hole in it, and new knowledge had made anaesthesia and intensive care more effective. There had been resources to put these to use for patients and for some of the most seriously ill the prospect of recovery had improved dramatically. But we also took satisfaction in knowing that, as it should be, our successors were much better trained than us, were capable of things we hadn't conceived of, were working in more challenging circumstances but seemed to be having just as good a time.

In July 2014 we attended a reunion for the staff of the Neurosurgical Unit from the 1970s. Sam was on great form. He spoke as ever without notes, warm, perceptive, witty, even hilarious. Time seemed to roll back.

Over the years we had talked about neurosurgery, not philosophy, but Sam gave me an enduring example of a powerful value system. I still use 'What would Sam think' as a personal yardstick. I felt his fundamental principles included that of 'non-exploitation of others'. He expressed this positively in selflessness, an acceptance of fellow humans and a driving ambition to make their lives better. Which he did many times over.

Sir Graham Teasdale

Lecturer, Department of Anatomy, 1967–69; Consultant Neurosurgeon, Institute of Neurological Sciences, Glasgow, 1975–2003; Professor and Head of Department of Neurosurgery, University of Glasgow, 1981–2003.

5

An Arresting Time in Texas

Gary Wilhelm

I met Sam Galbraith in the summer of 1976. He came to work at the Marine Biomedical Institute at the University of Texas Medical Branch, Galveston, Texas, where I was studying spinal root neuroanatomy under Professor Richard Coggeshall. Sam arrived at our lab with a very warm-looking wool suit speaking a language I could not understand: 'Guid morninmanames samyelgewbraitha'mfaeglesgaehoositgaun?' Later, I discovered he was speaking English. It took a while to understand his Scottish accent. I think that was the last day Sam wore a suit. We all were wearing T-shirts, jeans or Bermuda shorts.

We explained to Sam that we were expected to be at work from 7 a.m. – 8 at the latest. For the next year, he would saunter in between 9 and 10, complaining about starting work so early. Sam, at his epiglottal finest, greeted daily the visiting Japanese neurosurgeon in the lab. The two would mumble, smile and bow repeatedly. Later, after the visitor returned to Japan, Sam, with a fiendish sparkle in his eyes, admitted that he had always said: 'Guid mornin', Hirohito.' The Japanese surgeon had not understood a word. Sam took great delight in teasing and joking. So often, we laughed until we cried.

I gradually realised he was actually a neurosurgeon from Glasgow, Scotland. Sam blended into the lab immediately. We would usually walk home together each afternoon. We also shared lab space where he worked and I did small animal surgery. My attempts to operate on my bullfrogs and have them survive failed every time. I mentioned this to Sam and he said my surgical technique was terrible.

When I asked him to give me some help, he immediately began to teach me what I now know were good operative principles. He found some 4x4 gauze pads and soaked them with normal saline, placing them over the open wound and tissues. He taught me to handle the tissues 'with respect' and immediately my bullfrogs began to survive my surgical assaults. This was a key factor for me, since the animals had to survive to meet my experimental protocol. Many years later, I realised that Sam had been the only person in the lab trained as a surgeon.

One day Sam was watching me operate the Porter Blum MT-1 Ultramicrotome. He very casually said I did not seem to know much about ultramicrotomy. My thought was: 'What did he know?' He proceeded to show me over the next few days and weeks. As a result, I learned excellent ultramicrotomy technique from my new friend. I was cutting gold sections (the goal) in just a few weeks, with Sam's instruction. As it turned out, he really knew how to run an ultramicrotome as well and was a superb ultramicrotomist.

As I operated on another of the innumerable bullfrogs, Sam asked me about my religious beliefs. I told him I was a Lutheran. He said: 'Does that mean you're a Christian?', or something similar, and I said 'Yes.' He then stated, 'One cannot be a scientist and truly have a belief in God.' He added it did not make sense. I said it made sense to me. He said that was impossible. I said that I was doing it every day. We went back and forth about it several times. Suddenly, Sam stood up and said very firmly: 'This is impossible!' He then walked out of the lab and did not return until the next morning. He never brought it up again. It was only years later that I spoke to his Dad and found out his parents were devout evangelical Christians. Of course, Sam was not. Sam did joke with my wife, Kathy, and me about our annual Christmas cards, which I believe he always read but found humorous.

Sam visited my then girlfriend (now my wife of 37 years), Katherine Kuhlman Wilhelm, in San Antonio one weekend. Sam and I both flew up to central Texas on Southwest Airlines. It was $50 for a round trip at the time. Kathy was a first lieutenant in the US Army Nurse Corps and was assigned to Brooke Army Medical Center. We both remember Sam saying our American breakfast toast was too moist. He went around Kathy's kitchen propping up pieces of toast here and there to allow them to dry out, since we did not have a 'proper' toast rack.

Kathy and I also made pancakes that weekend. We argued over who was actually in charge of making the pancakes. For months afterwards, Sam would often say out of the blue: 'I am making the pancakes!' imitating our little argument over who was actually in charge of pancake operation that day.

Just before Sam left to return to Glasgow, he and Jim Rose, a neurosurgeon at the University of Texas, were drinking beer by Sam's apartment swimming pool on a Sunday afternoon. I was not there, but evidently they went through quite a few cans of beer. Jim left and Sam was still by the pool. The next morning, Sam was not at the lab. He had never missed a day. I asked and was told Sam was in the Galveston jail. Jim Rose went down and bailed him out. The police had arrested Sam thinking he was a drunken sailor from one of Galveston's ships in the harbour due to his accent. Sam told me his jailors kept asking him what he did for a living. He told them they would never believe him if he told the truth.

My wife, Kathy, and I were able to visit Sam in Glasgow, and later both Sam and Nicola in Glasgow over the years. Once, Sam took us to the 'hut', which I think was owned by the Scottish Mountaineering Club. Earlier in the day, Kathy had purchased a traditional 'Scottish Bun Cake', which Sam stated, with some disgust, was only purchased by tourists. When we got to the hut, there was no food there and no electricity. It was around midnight and Sam started a fire in the fireplace. I think we may have had a beer or two or some Scotch. As we were sitting there, Sam said, 'Hey, do you still have that Scottish Bun Cake?' We shared it that night! There was nothing left.

On another occasion, we were with Sam at a pub in Glasgow. I remember asking him how they came up with the Glasgow Coma Scale. He said there were too many practitioners in the countryside sending patients to their neurosurgery department who were supposed to be 'in coma', but then arrived walking and talking into their clinic. The scale was to allow the neurosurgeons to know who was truly comatose. I persisted, asking, 'But how did you develop the process?' Sam said, with a mischievous twinkle in his eye, 'The coma scale was developed on the back of a napkin in a pub.' Sam explained that in Scotland there was always time for 'lateral thinking', and that Americans spent too much time working way too hard, never allowing time for any creative processing. Now that I am an old physician, I believe Sam was correct about my country's lack of lateral thinking.

On our second visit in 1986, Sam looked wasted and gaunt with no temporal fat pads. What had happened? Sam set up a projector in his living room and showed us slides from his trip to Nepal with several members of the Scottish Mountaineering Club. The plan had been to climb an unclimbed peak. Before the ascent, a blizzard that night kept the group busy clearing wet, heavy snow off their tent so they would not suffocate. By next morning, Sam's friend Sandy Reid was hypothermic. Even with another warmer person next to him in his sleeping bag, Sandy kept shivering. Sam realised that Sandy would die without help, so he and a Sherpa descended to get help in carrying Sandy off the mountain. This event had deeply shaken Sam. He seemed to be re-evaluating everything about his life since he and his group had come close to dying. An Indian army unit had all perished that same night, found dead in their tents. Sam had saved his friend's life, yet Sandy still died before Sam, of heart disease in 2013.

Kathy and I visited Sam in London when he was an MP. He gave us a tour around Parliament and got us great gallery seats for Prime Minister's Questions. Earlier that day, Sam took us to a room with large leather chairs and couches. He, Kathy and I all fell asleep sitting in this room. Every now and then, other MPs would drift in and out of the room which overlooked the River Thames. All I could think was, how did two farm kids from Ohio end up taking a nap with a Scottish neurosurgeon who is an MP in the private rooms of the UK Parliament? It was solely due to Sam and his unfailing friendship.

The last time we saw Sam and Nicola was in 1991 in Glasgow. Kathy had just returned from her combat deployment to the first Gulf War as an army nurse anaesthetist. Mhairi had been born and we got to meet her on that visit. Sam was truly a changed man and obviously in love with his little daughter. I was amazed to hear him sing 'The wheels on the bus go round and round' over and over. It seemed light years from our days in Galveston, but it had been only fifteen years. Of course, Sam by then was a single lung transplant survivor, but this never seemed to get him down. I remember he did say that his anti-rejection medications would turn his 'nuts to cellulose'. I guess he overcame this, since he eventually had three daughters.

Now and then, I tell someone I knew the group that wrote up the Glasgow Coma Scale and that I had met Graham Teasdale, one of its authors. I get quite a few 'Really?' sort of looks. Sometimes, I can hardly believe it is true myself.

It was so much fun to be with Sam and I am glad I had the chance. He was an original. Although Sam was firm that he was not a Christian and not a believer, I often thought he was one of the most thoughtful, kind, Christian-like people I have known. He genuinely cared about others and showed it in his thoughtfulness and manner. I do miss him.

Gary B. Wilhelm

Graduate PhD Student, Marine Biomedical Institute, Galveston, Texas, 1976–77; Colonel and Flight Surgeon, US Army.

With acknowledgement for input from Lauren A. Langford, Research Medical Student, Marine Biological Institute, 1976–7; Jim Rose, Neurosurgeon, University of Texas Medical Branch, 1977; and Katherine Jean Wilhelm.

6

A Pied Piper We Were Happy
to Follow

Alistair Jenkins

Occasionally in neurosurgery, a case goes better than you expected, and you're out of theatre with a little time on your hands. Although, as always, there was a massive pile of paperwork lurking menacingly in my office, I turned to the ENT surgeon and the registrar operating with me and said 'Bike ride . . . ?'

Forty minutes later we were buzzing through the lanes with that wonderful guilty feeling you get when you have managed to dog off work on the best day of summer. As I often do, I thought of Sam and his perpetual motto: 'Work hard, play hard.'

Sam did both, and then some. He was the outstanding graduate of his year, and had an intimidating list of publications; but he was also an accomplished and prolific climber, and a – well, enthusiastic – skier and runner. His application to the art of drinking was already legendary by the time I met him: he held court in the Aragon pub on Byres Road most Fridays, and many students fell under his spell there. I wasn't one of these, and it wasn't till I very reluctantly turned up at the Institute of Neurological Sciences for a rotational stint in neurosurgery in 1981 that I came any closer to him than the auditorium of a lecture theatre.

I was dreading that job. My undergraduate career had been very enjoyable but my involvement in actual medical studies had been somewhat tangential. Having, as I saw it, blagged my way through my house jobs, I was finally going to come unstuck on the cold hard facts of neurology, and my planned career as a maybe-orthopaedic-maybe-general surgeon would require some revision. But it didn't turn out like that: neurosurgery is logical and proved fascinating and compelling; almost immediately, I was hooked and managed to cope with the SHO post – the most junior of junior jobs in neurosurgery.

At that point I didn't work directly with Sam, but he seemed to be omnipresent: encouraging, cajoling and hectoring in theatre; being the first – always the first – to spot an inconsistency in a presentation at the academic meetings, and announce it loudly; slumped in his characteristic position in a chair at the back of the X-ray conferences, legs akimbo and only his spine in contact with the seat, giving someone just enough rope and then saying: 'That's a load of bollocks!' – a saying to be branded, much later and in a very different environment, as 'unparliamentary'!

Sam could be rude. Very rude. In those days it was still common for people to ask, 'Do you mind if I smoke?' and Sam had a stock answer: 'Certainly. Do you mind if I fart?' But as a true socialist, he was rude to everyone, senior or junior, male or female. And somehow he always got away with it – mostly because there was never an ounce of malice in it. One of the extraordinary things about Sam was that in spite of the politics and the potential rivalries in the hothouse of neurosurgery, and his uncompromising approach to these, nobody disliked him. Similarly, he seemed to dislike nobody, however forthrightly he might criticise them, and he had an affectionate nickname for everyone – usually one which showed his ability to see very rapidly the essence of their personality.

Sam encouraged me to continue in neurosurgery. It felt to me an enormous privilege to have his approval and I returned as a proper trainee in 1984, working – and playing – with Sam until he left just over three years later.

In the mid-1980s the Institute was a very demanding place in which to work: a united front was seen as all-important, and this contributed to the international standing of the Unit. Sam was the ideal ambassador at conferences, strong and dogmatic but with erudition and humour. While occasionally an episode of over-refreshment the previous evening could detract from his performance, with Graham Teasdale he was responsible for maintaining and increasing the prominence of Glasgow on the neurosurgical scene that their mentor Bryan Jennett had established. So when any of the junior surgeons had a paper to present at such a meeting, they were ruthlessly rehearsed by Sam beforehand. As well as the scientific content, the language was mercilessly analysed for repetition, tautology, and in particular for using a 'fancy' word or phrase when a plain one would do. This became ingrained in all of us; I find myself now passing this on to my own trainees. Why, indeed, use the terms 'upper limb' or 'verbalising', when 'arm' and 'talking' are not only shorter but more easily understood?

Conciseness was also the essence of Sam's operating. All unnecessary fuss was avoided. An aneurysm was there to be clipped, not toyed with, and his operations were a joy to watch. Quick, precise and accurate, he displayed the single most important hallmark of the virtuoso: he made it look easy. He coaxed and cajoled us into trying to emulate him and to varying levels we succeeded – but we never equalled his flair and panache. Teaching at that time was all done by example rather than instruction and in this Sam excelled – though his formal lectures were also hugely enjoyable (and not very formal).

Ward rounds were expected to start exactly on time, and Sam would set off – sometimes alone – exactly at the specified time. An extremely caring doctor, his bedside manner was unorthodox: he would often stand with one foot on the patient's bed, and the exchange rarely lasted more than a minute. But of course when the day ended he was usually to be found back in the ward talking with those same patients. What a contrast his upbeat chats were to today's perception of the way to talk to patients, hedged with caveats, excuses and politically-correct verbiage. As with his operating, he managed to instil absolute confidence in the patient – a confidence which was never misplaced – while lacing his talk with humour and empathy. A common feature of surgical rounds is the 'board round', or quick visual check of the patients. On one such occasion he stood at the door of a patient's cubicle – a slightly hard-of-hearing lady with an aneurysm of the basilar artery – and announced: 'She's the basilar!'

'WHAT did he call me??' she demanded, as Sam swept off.

The great thing about being Sam's trainee was that he genuinely looked on the juniors as his friends. A very short time after joining the Unit, I was meeting him regularly at his flat in Partickhill early on a Saturday morning, ready for a day's hill-walking, ice-climbing, or skiing. That flat . . . always stiflingly hot, with the only decoration climbing ropes of various colours, and a rather fetching bust of Lenin. And, of course, books: lots of them, *Das Kapital* rubbing shoulders with *The Rights of Man* and Northfield's *Surgery of the Central Nervous System*. Sam had the rather disconcerting habit of answering the door with nothing on whatsoever, so at least the bust of Lenin gave us something to look at while he dressed. On one occasion, to our relief, he was wearing a white towelling dressing gown – but unfortunately a cord was not part of the outfit, and the effect was somewhat spoiled.

Sam was a sort of Pied Piper figure and we never refused the opportunity to follow him. He would bark out orders: 'Dorothy – you take the sandwiches; Alistair – you take the ropes.' Mystified foreign registrars would be swept along on the easier trips and never failed to be stunned by Scotland's scenery. I remember two, who had never seen snow before, rolling around in it and joyfully throwing snowballs at the top of a climb in Glencoe.

On all these excursions, as in everything, Sam exuded ability, confidence – and midge repellent. In the cramped confines of his overheated and hermetically sealed Golf GTI (not an elitist car, he protested: 'Nothing, but nothing, is too good for the workers') we rattled along the narrow Loch Lomond road in all weathers, usually to Glencoe, never missing a stop at the Drovers Inn on the way back to refuel with a whisky, hot chocolate and a toastie. Often this would be topped off later by a visit to the Ashoka, Sam's favourite curry house.

One winter's day it had snowed heavily overnight, and Sam and I thought it a good idea to ski to work. Unfortunately we only had downhill skis, and only the first few hundred yards were actually downhill. There was also the small matter of the Clyde Tunnel, where curiously no snow had fallen and through which we had to lug our skis. Nevertheless we trudged on through Govan, where skis were a bit of a novelty, and got to the Institute about mid-morning. None of our colleagues managed to get to work that day.

It was while skiing at Aviemore with Sam one day that I first noticed his odd breathing pattern – when out of breath after a run, he would pant like a dog rather than take deep breaths. I thought nothing of it. He went off some time later to the Himalayas, and on return had obviously lost weight and was looking older. From then on, things got rapidly worse, and eventually his diagnosis became clear. He had developed fibrosing alveolitis, as his sister had some years before.

By that time he had left neurosurgery for a career in politics. While we all knew how passionately he believed in fairness and justice, we were shocked that he could turn his back on a profession which he clearly loved and at which he excelled. However as he was standing in a safe Tory seat in a posh suburb we assumed he had no chance – as did Sam. A few days before the election, however, he said to me: 'I think I might win this!' – and of course he did, with a sizeable majority.

Becoming an MP is a little like going to prison – it starts immediately and Sam had gone almost before we realised. Surgically, academically and educationally, he left a massive gap, but more importantly the Institute lost a vital part of its spirit, and we trainees lost a mentor and role model. The break was absolute: though at first he operated abroad during the parliamentary recess, I never saw him operate again.

Sam went on to an equally distinguished career in politics, though he would surely have achieved even more were it not for his illness. I saw him in hospital just before his transplant. He was clearly on his last legs, but an appropriate donor lung became available and he had his operation in Newcastle. His recovery was surprisingly rapid; I knew he was really on the mend when he started being rude to me again. Twenty-four years later he was the longest surviving lung recipient, and we all thought that he would live forever . . .

Sam would not like a eulogy. He hated pomposity, and I never heard him once boast about his abilities in any sphere. He would probably be astonished if he knew how often I think, 'What would Sam do?', and even more surprised that the question extends to so many areas outside medicine.

If you see me limping, it's because of an accident I had when I was climbing some practice rocks and fell off. When I was in hospital, Sam teased me mercilessly. I never told him that the reason I was doing it was so I could keep up with him.

If you see me struggling in theatre, it's for the same reason.

Alistair Jenkins

Neurosurgical Trainee, Glasgow, 1981–82, 1984–88; Consultant Neurosurgeon, Newcastle, 1990 continuing.

7

Nurses Saw a Charismatic
Team Player

Margaret Harkess

In the Institute of Neurological Sciences in the 1970s there was a group of six distinguished neurosurgeons, led by Mr Alistair Paterson and Professor Bryan Jennett.

Their skills and interests were different, and the theatre staff took great pride in looking after 'their' consultants, so the ethos of team-work was strong and was encouraged.

It was a formal work-place: full titles were the order of the day amongst all grades of staff. The theatre staff were dedicated neurosurgery nurses, so we became very knowledgeable about our specialities, and in certain instances were able to contribute our skills to assist the surgeons position their patients correctly for surgery, act as first assistant, or give advice to a junior registrar struggling with venous bleeding before he had to call the on-call consultant.

So in 1974, into this august arena came Mr Galbraith to commence neurosurgical training. Within five years he had become a consultant, but this didn't change his personality or his unique, inimitable style. A charismatic presence – irrepressible – he bucked the myth that surgeons were 'proper'! He asked questions, he demanded answers; he ruffled feathers; he challenged practice. He was by turns outrageous, provoking, irritating, hugely entertaining, compassionate and caring; blunt and uncompromising. And above all, he was a really good surgeon. Everyone enjoyed working with and for him.

The registrars did a lot of the work at night in those days. If

47

you were the scrub nurse on call when Sam was the receiving surgeon, you could be fairly sure that nothing unnecessary would be brought into theatre. This was before the compulsory use of seat belts in cars (1981) so there were some very messy trauma cases – victims of road traffic accidents – where you spent time just fishing out the shards of windscreen glass embedded in the patient's face and scalp, and suturing the many lacerations after the head injury had been dealt with.

Neurosurgery, for the surgeon, is probably one of the loneliest of specialities. There is only a very confined space in which to work, the help the assistant can provide is very limited, the scrub nurse is there to provide instrumentation; but the ultimate success or failure of an operation lies with the lead surgeon. Their strengths and frailties are exposed, there in the raw. The mental and physical stamina required to deal with unforeseen problems and rise above them is extreme. How a surgeon reacts and responds to such incidents is almost a make or break for that individual. Scrub nurses and floor staff recognise the surgeons' abilities very quickly, and on such assessments is the delivery of assistance intuitively decided. Sam stood up to that scrutiny unfazed. He was a natural leader and a great team player, so in the surgical environment, Sam had the total commitment of the theatre staff behind him.

On the daily work-board, you looked to see where your allocation was going to be, and depending on which theatre you had been assigned to, there might or might not be a mental sigh of resignation when you saw which surgeon was operating!

The initials S.L.G. identified Sam's presence in the operating department – on his theatre boots with yellow anti-static strips down the backs; on his box of 'special' instruments that he liked to have available for whatever procedure he was involved with; or his 'own' perforator and burr, kept as sharp as possible. In those days, only consultants got to use power drills to open a skull! The registrars had to make do with a Hudson brace, perforator and burr, followed by a Gigli saw in order to raise a bone flap. If the perforator or burr was blunt, it made for a lot of extra effort and frustration on the surgeon's part. So, as the scrub nurse, if you knew that there was a nice sharp burr and perforator sitting sterile on a shelf, they were pulled into use. Then there would much growling from Sam, 'Have those bloody registrars been using my stuff again?'

Sam was such a unique person. Really, he defies description. He was a truly genuine person, who cared passionately about the NHS and its total worth to the populace. So he was outspoken in his opinions regarding private healthcare. He kept everyone grounded in theatre: no-one was allowed to have a huge ego; if there was a surfacing of self-importance, it took just a sly comment and the status quo would be restored.

On the wards his informal approach was a breath of fresh air to nurses and patients alike, who were used to medical staff being very formal. He was great fun, as he loved a laugh and enjoyed teasing the nurses. One girl who arrived on the ward as a young staff nurse wasn't used to Sam's wicked sense of humour. He soon realised that it was really easy to make her blush, and she became a regular target of his quick wit. Then he discovered that she held strong feminist views, so he called her Mrs Pankhurst! Phoning the ward to discuss something with her, he asked for Mrs Pankhurst, but was informed that there was no patient of that name in the ward!

Patients loved and respected him because he spoke with and to them at their level. When he was the bearer of bad news, Sam would go to see the patient on his own, sit on their bed and speak gently and quietly with them. Weekend ward rounds are less formal, but Sam took 'dress down' to a new level. His idea of casual was a disreputable brown woollen jersey, with large holes in the elbows. So he would wander round, seeing his patients, helping himself to their grapes on the way.

He was kind enough to bring in sausages, bacon and rolls for ward staff, and would sit and eat with them, enjoying the easy camaraderie. However, the Unit senior nurse was soon on the warpath to put a stop to this practice. It was deemed a bit unfair to the patients, who had the tantalising aroma of cooking bacon and sausages wafting through the ward but were not able to partake as well.

Sam was Sam to everyone. He was easy to talk to and with. The staff found an empathetic ear for their grievances over their pay. So when COHSE (Confederation of Health Service Employees) organised a nationwide demonstration and 24-hour strike in 1982, Sam was a major supporter and headed the march in Aberdeen. For this deed, the Health Board withheld half a day's salary. Undeterred, Sam declined to take the full value of a 10 per cent pay rise to doctors when other staff were awarded only 4 per cent and donated the difference to an NHS hospital. For that he was even more of a hero to the staff!

The theatre coffee room was always a good arena for debate! There was an almost palpable fizz in the air when Sam would wander in, briefly scan whoever was assembled there, give a throw-away comment to see if anyone would take the bait; ask a pertinent question, whatever, there was always dialogue of some description when he was around.

He would tease the theatre staff to the total disapproval of the sister in charge, who would remonstrate with him, but often to little avail. One scrub nurse newly returned to work after a holiday abroad was assisting Sam, but failing to keep pace with him. 'Come on, do you think you're still lying out there, topless in the sun?'

Seeing a very heavily pregnant member of staff coming in for her night shift, he gazed at her in horror and pleaded: 'Oh Christ – see and don't cough!' Staff never took offence at these utterances.

He was no respecter of race or creed: his own colleagues were not immune to his indiscriminate wit. An experienced neurosurgeon from overseas – but not very fluent in English on his arrival at the Institute – was assisting Sam at a surgical procedure, and totally accepted Sam's instruction that when he was ready to stitch up and close the wound, he should ask the scrub nurse for a 's----t'. That man's English improved *very* quickly.

Awaiting an anaesthetist's presence in theatre for a surgical procedure, Sam was asked if he had seen the person in question at all. 'Oh yes,' he replied, 'he's coming along the corridor being chased by a tortoise, and the tortoise is winning.'

Remembrances of Sam are many and so varied. The nursing staff just loved him to bits, he'd been everyone's brother or son; so there was a great sense of loss when he left the Institute to become an MP at Westminster.

And he continued to impact on our emotions. There was the sense of pride when he appeared on TV – he was one of 'our' boys; we felt huge concern over his transplant, and relief at his recovery; and we shared the happiness as the years and achievements just went on and on.

In February 2011, I was attending the memorial service of a former colleague, and happened to meet up with Graham Teasdale and Sam. After the service, we made our way to a hotel for refreshments and to chat to other Institute colleagues. We were sitting, gently reminiscing on times past, when Sam commented, reflectively, that it was 'really important to keep the pages turning, backwards and forwards; to remember . . .'

Margaret Harkess

Charge Nurse in the Neurosurgical Theatres, Institute of Neurological Sciences, Glasgow, 1973–2009.

Grateful acknowledgements to other colleagues for their input: Margaret C. Ritchie, Diane Fraser, Lynn Watson, Lynne Leonard.

8

My Personal Life-Saver and Political Inspiration

Torcuil Crichton

Sam Galbraith, who lived a remarkably long time given his odds, was a big figure in my life.

Most Scottish political journalists would have come across Galbraith as the gruff, no-nonsense member of Donald Dewar's Scottish Office team who remained by his side as Labour's lost leader moved his operation from Westminster to open the first Scottish Parliament.

I knew him then, and still chuckle at the irreverence and intelligence he brought to the job of politics in the early days of Holyrood. But my first encounter with Sam Galbraith was years beforehand. I met him in 1976 when he was a neurosurgeon in the team that treated me at the Southern General hospital for a serious head injury. He saved my life.

Perhaps I shouldn't have gone back upstairs that February Monday morning for one final check on the condition of my Airfix Russian infantry, but such things are a high priority for an 11-year-old in a rush. I never made it back down, at least not using the steps. My mother found me in a crumpled heap at the bottom of the staircase in our croft house, bleeding and drifting in and out of consciousness. My injuries were obviously severe and there was no way I could be treated at the local hospital in Stornoway on the Isle of Lewis. Later in the day a decision was taken to lift me by air ambulance to the Southern General Hospital in Glasgow where I could be assessed and operated on.

I was there for over three weeks. The Southern General's CT scanner – one of the first in the country – was pressed into service, lumbar punctures were administered, it was the NHS at its glorious best.

Compared to other young patients in ward 64 who were in mortal danger, I was lucky. There was no brain injury, but the lining around the brain was torn and I needed to be patched up. The team that operated was led by Professor Bryan Jennett who had established Glasgow as a world centre for neurosurgery and made major advances in the care and management of patients with head injuries.

But for my anguished parents it was the skill and personal touch of the younger surgeon on the team, Sam Galbraith, that were a great comfort. For a young boy in a turban of bandages, he was simply a hero.

That should have been it, but the procedure wasn't a success the first time and it was Galbraith himself, several months later, who saw me for a follow-up and performed a second operation. That meant another shaved head and bandages for me, but ever afterwards Sam's name, as the one who had fixed me properly, was revered in our household.

He wasn't there at the Southern General seven years later when my young brother went one better than me and fell head-first off a cliff near home. By then our family knew the awful routine: air ambulance, Southern General, ward 64. But that's another story, which my brother lived to tell.

Spool forwards to late 1982, and as a first-year student at Glasgow University I bumped into Sam Galbraith again on the corner of Byres Road. The Falklands War had been won, and despite a recession the Tory government was guaranteed re-election although we couldn't admit that to ourselves, so the fight went on. There he was alone, with a megaphone battery-box slung over his shoulder, campaigning to protect the NHS from Thatcherite cuts. In hindsight it might seem like a futile protest. He cut a solitary figure, slightly stooped even then. But the voice, amplified through the loudhailer, was unmistakable and what he spoke about was very important.

I approached and introduced myself and, remarkably, he remembered me.

I'd just started becoming politicised myself, but somehow in my naivety I had no idea that surgeons could be political too or, even better, that they could be against Margaret Thatcher. But then, everyone in the West of Scotland seemed to be against Margaret Thatcher as that long decade of Tory rule spun out into the next one.

Political activism in Scotland at that time was not viewed through the prism of nationalism as it is now and the discourse was not so parochial or inward-looking. The strength of the trade union movement and the left meant that internationalism was a strong strand in politics. As students we would have serious discussions in the pub about the Sandinistas and whether it was practical to do something to resist the United States' stranglehold.

Older and more committed people like Sam Galbraith and Brian Wilson were doing so much more, crossing the Atlantic to report on the Nicaraguan revolution and raising something like £60,000 through Scottish Medical Aid for Nicaragua.

By then I'd heard that Galbraith was a keen mountaineer and had him down as a Dougal Haston kind of figure, the legendary Scottish climbing pioneer, off in the far Himalaya when not in the operating theatre.

Next, I met him in the late '80s, by which time Brian Wilson had recruited me to become a journalist on the *West Highland Free Press* on Skye. It was on a road trip down from Broadford to Glasgow that Brian mentioned his first stop in the city would be at an anti-apartheid rally in the city being hosted by Sam Galbraith. I know that guy, I said, so off we headed to the reception (it could have been in the old SOGAT offices on Clyde Street) and met up. And that is how I was recruited to the Anti-Apartheid Movement. I think I still have the 'Free Mandela' mug.

When he became a Labour MP, and later an MSP and Minister in Holyrood, I was a national journalist reporting on politics. Sam was the right kind of politician for Scotland, rooted in working class sensibilities with the confidence and education to take on the Civil Service machine and any opponent who crossed his path. The gruff Greenock accent, the sharp wit and intelligence went down a storm in the early days of the Holyrood Parliament. He was the master of repartee and the instant put-down. His bark, I'm assured, was worse than his bite.

His bedside manner helped too. Having a parent and a medic in charge of the school system was an assurance to voters. But as Education Minister he faced a crisis when the Scottish Qualifications Authority messed up the Higher exam results in August 2000. Parents were up in arms. Things looked pretty bad for the Dewar administration. Sam popped up on television in a clip recorded on the Isle of Lewis where he was on summer holiday with his family. I suspect the questions were read out by the single camera operator, Ged Yeats, on location rather than posed by an interrogative reporter down the line. Galbraith did not pass up on the open goal.

On television that night no one was more outraged than the Education Minister. The situation was a disgrace, people were right to be angry, no one more angry than the person ultimately responsible. As a lesson in political distraction and distancing it was a masterclass, but once the crisis had passed Sam was relieved to be moved on from the education brief with his reputation intact.

His last intervention in politics came at the time of the

Scottish referendum in 2014. He re-emerged into public life to tell his own story about how the British NHS had kept him alive when he was days from death: 'I was just another British person in Newcastle. There were other Scots folk there and they were all treated the same,' he said, recalling the life-saving lung operation. 'There were no forms to fill in, no money to be considered. It was all just done because people needed it done. I fear for that under a separate Scotland.' His intervention was timely, because it was testament to the campaigning skill of the nationalists that they were working overtime to turn one of the biggest threats from independence, the disintegration of the NHS, into an argument in their favour by putting about the lie that the NHS was in danger from staying within the UK, due to Tory market reforms. Sam magisterially pointed out that Holyrood was completely empowered to do things differently in Scotland. He might have added that this was in no small measure due to his own dedicated efforts.

When Sam made his intervention in the *Daily Record* I wrote a small commentary, reminding those who were too young to know and others who might have forgotten just who he was. I used the experience of my own encounters with Sam at various stages in my life, just as I've told you now, to explain why it was this medic's voice that was the one to be trusted.

'Having fought his own illness, he's back with a serious message about the consequences of independence,' I wrote. 'No matter what side of the debate you are on, his is a voice that demands attention and respect. Sam Galbraith, when he was done saving my life and countless others, campaigned for the right causes all through my life.'

Torcuil Crichton

Patient, Neurosurgical Department, Institute of Neurological Sciences, Glasgow, 1976; Westminster Editor, *Daily Record*, 2010 continuing.

9

Leisure and Recreation

David Hamilton

Leisure was important to Sam and brought out his talents and his determination: when his energies were curbed later, he made adjustments to suit. I first met him when I arrived at the Western Infirmary Professorial Surgical Unit in 1971 and I saw Professor Kay and his entourage being taken round his wards at speed by a young sharp-eyed junior who ignored any delaying unhelpful comments from the others. At the end of the week, I suggested that we have a pint together in the Aragon pub in Byres Road adjacent to the hospital. From then on we shared much, including our leisure time. The Aragon was the regular Friday night meeting place for most of that group of young Western Infirmary surgeons later to be 'Truants', i.e. making their contributions in many other fields rather than clinical surgery.

Sam's early sporting interest was in football, playing in the back green of the tenement block in Greenock. In his early secondary school years at Greenock High School he played the game at right back and had the usual youthful ambition to play football for Scotland: this was shelved when he realised that, at that time, his birth in England excluded him. In later school years he took up rowing, organised locally by the Deputy Rector at Greenock's Royal West Amateur Boat Club (founded 1866) on the Clyde shore.

Soon he started travelling to Glasgow on Saturdays for the four- or eight-man 'shell' boat rowing on the Clyde at Glasgow Green using the boats of the Glasgow Printing Trade Amateur

Rowing Club – whose members were probably not welcome at the Henley Regatta since they worked with their hands during the week. This club was located next door to the University's Glasgow Argonauts club, who were more acceptable in polite rowing circles. His recreational rowing on the Clyde near Greenock continued and might include a stay-over on Saturdays with friends in a cave on the Kilcreggan shore opposite Greenock, where they got up to no good. He was active in the local Scouts and, showing talent and leadership, gained rapid promotion to Scout Leader and the highest award of Queen's Scout.

At Glasgow University, Sam's energies went into his studies and he largely dropped his hobbies and sport. This changed about 1975 during a spell when he worked at the Belford Hospital in Fort William. Brother Roderick was climbing on Ben Nevis nearby and took Sam along. The family had always enjoyed hill-walking and camping, led by their father, but Sam was soon smitten with rock-climbing and the sport became an important challenge to him. His interest in climbing chimed in well with his left-wing sympathies, since the Clyde shipyard workers had a tradition, dating from the Depression, of staying in bothies in Glen Coe, and living off the land (and the landowners' beasts). Climbing was not a gentleman's preserve in Scotland. The gentlemen did have their elite Scottish Mountaineering Club, originally limited to Alpinists, but Sam later made the grade and was elected to the Club. Sam's love of the outdoors and his hopes for reform of land ownership in Scotland meant that he was tasked with bringing to the Commons (with Brian Wilson) the first attempt to create National Parks in Scotland. His National Parks (Scotland) Bill was introduced by Sam in 1996, predictably opposed by the Tories and the Scottish landowners. The Bill stood no chance of success, but Sam had put down a marker for the future and the establishment of the Parks had to await the arrival of the Scottish Parliament.

The Friday night Aragon gathering was well established early on, and the core members of our group for many years were Sam, Sandy Reid (later an academic pathologist in Edinburgh, dying in 2013), myself, Harry Burns and Andrew Bradley. The discourse was what is now called 'progressive' and the link between poverty and ill health was a given. Occasionally new young trainees (or professors) would join our group and express sympathies with the Conservative Party: they did not last long. Sam and Sandy now climbed regularly on weekends off and the rest of us could ski: steadily the Friday night companionship extended into regular winter weekend visits to the Spey Valley. Soon we took cottages with long lets over the winter, sharing the modest cost as a syndicate, and we headed north on Friday nights after sorting out the world's problems first in the Aragon. The climbers climbed in the Cairngorm corries and the rest of us skied. The weather could be adverse and lack of snow or high winds or both was common, but this was no problem since the convivial Spey Valley was famous as a non-skiing skiing centre: Sam and Sandy might also have an enjoyable non-climbing climbing weekend.

Up north, with tongues loosened in our favourite pubs, grand schemes emerged as we put the world to rights, designing an ideal society with the idealism of youth. This free-ranging dialectic continued over mince and potatoes and red wine back at the cottage. One non-intellectual challenge was that we often had no corkscrew. Sam, as a brain surgeon, was given the task of getting the cork out with a knife and fork. As a pragmatic, speedy operator, he preferred the nuclear option of hitting the neck of the bottle sharply on the edge of the china sink.

Others were free to join us, as were visitors to Glasgow, and over time our future wives joined the group. The new professor of surgery at Oxford joined us once. He was given what we liked to call the best bedroom, one which had some warmth, being next to the living room and its fire in the tiny cottage. After he retired to bed, the wide-ranging debate continued as usual. Sam and Sandy had an epiphany in the small hours, namely that people should not own any property, but hold everything in common. Ever practical, we sought specific examples and proposals. No toothbrushes, it was agreed, should be owned. All toothbrushes should be held in common and should be awaiting everyone everywhere and on any travels. The bemused Oxford surgeon, unable to sleep, should have been familiar with the general drift of this utopian philosophy, but emerged at breakfast to ask, 'What the ---- was all that about toothbrushes?'

After these weekends, going back down the road, and at other times, we had another gathering for many years on Sunday nights at a pub near the Sick Children's Hospital, thereafter moving down the road to the Ashoka Indian restaurant nearby, where we often got the big table in the basement. If any life events were current, we would plan ahead and celebrate with a feast based on a marinated roasted leg of lamb, ordered 48 hours ahead.

But as we got older and involved with tough decisions in the real world, even Sam, heading towards a political career, became quite pragmatic. The discussions now included 'the Scottish Question', previously seen by Sam as only one small part of the worldwide struggle by the working masses against the ruling classes. Only Sandy kept the faith and the pure socialist line. Sam even dropped his hostility to bourgeois skiing, purchasing the gear and using it occasionally. We also had some European ski resort chalet trips and jousted with the uncomprehending Sloane Ranger chalet girls.

In later life, when retired and with his exercise tolerance down, in summer another hobby emerged, which needed only walking at a gentle pace in his beloved outdoors. He was a well-respected member of the Clyde and Argyll Fungus group, who in addition to their meetings, made planned surveys of areas of interest, often in remote areas, and he, like the others, would return to classify unusual species by microscopy. He had a personal niche interest. His long-lasting lung transplant was functioning by courtesy of cyclosporine – a powerful anti-rejection fungal extract.

Sam also conceded that golf had its attractions and started to play regularly at the Strathclyde University course at Ross Priory, and also at the public Knightswood course near home – 'Royal Knightswood' as he christened it. By then he was a medical member in the Scottish Tribunals Service dealing with disability claims, and was concerned to find that his fellow weekday players were often on state benefits awarded for their inability to walk.

Returning to an old haunt, Sam and Nicola bought a chalet at Newtonmore in the Spey Valley in 2012. There he could play golf on the flat local course, and visits to the rough might be rewarded by fungal finds. When he visited us in St Andrews he enjoyed a round, latterly using a buggy, but at the 19th hole there was the constraint that sadly his cyclosporine medication interacted with whisky and gave him a headache.

On one occasion earlier when we lunched at the Royal and Ancient Golf Club, we encountered an old medical friend, a well-known, very deaf, Glasgow Tory R&A member who still had political ambitions. In the staid Big Room of the Club, Sam greeted him and had to shout. 'Now that New Labour is in, your chance of a knighthood has gone!' he loudly teased the Tory. The members' gin and tonics rattled a bit.

Sam had a passion for life and living: he used his leisure to the full.

David Hamilton

Lecturer, later Consultant, Department of Surgery, Western Infirmary, Glasgow, 1971–2004.

10

These Were His Mountains

Andrew Bradley

Sam was uncharacteristically silent as he contemplated the enormity of what lay ahead. Having just completed a rising traverse across a steep sheet of snow-ice, he inserted a long ice-screw into the ice slope and clipped into it the ropes that stretched between us. Before readying myself to climb, I took a photograph of him perched in the shadow of the snow-covered rocks. This turned out by chance to be a powerful climbing image and was, many years later, submitted to the Scottish Mountaineering Club to accompany Sam's obituary.

We were poised to begin the ascent of Point Five Gully, a 300-metre vertical ice climb on the north face of Ben Nevis. I climbed up to join Sam, and then continued past him before pausing under a bulging wall of blue ice – the first major crux of the route. The ropes provided considerable psychological comfort, but whether, if either of us slipped, they would have stopped us falling or simply catapulted each of us in turn to the corrie floor far below remained thankfully unknown. Point Five Gully was without any doubt the most serious winter climb either of us had attempted and we were by no means confident of success.

By any reckoning Point Five Gully is a serious winter climb, with no prospect of escape to easier terrain and a reputation for spindrift avalanches. The unimaginatively named route had acquired legendary status and climbing it had been a long-standing ambition of ours. Our expedition had started the previous

evening when we drove up from Glasgow in Sam's recently purchased car.

From Fort William we had followed the rugged path that
ascends alongside the tumbling waters of the Allt a'Mhuilinn.
Sam was a proud member of the Scottish Mountaineering Club
and this gave us access to the CIC (Charles Inglis Clark) Memorial Hut, a climber's sanctuary situated under the North Face of
Ben Nevis. We rose early to a freezing morning, and headed up
towards the great North East Buttress. The entire mountain was
heavily encrusted with ice and there was no place on earth that
we would rather have been.

Sam had, in his teenage years, developed a deep love of the
Scottish mountains, cherishing the chance to be among them
whenever possible. Like many other youngsters his passion for
Scottish climbing had been fuelled by the evocative literature
that captured so well the essence and romanticism of Scottish
climbing; books like *Mountaineering in Scotland* and *Undiscovered Scotland* written by W.H. Murray in the 1940s, but timeless
in their power to fire the imagination.

It was while studying medicine at Glasgow University that
Sam's mountain-climbing experience had really taken off. As a
student and then a young doctor he climbed with fellow medics
and close friends Sandy Reid and Ewan Macdonald, and they, in
turn, became part of a ragged bunch of Glasgow-based climbers known affectionately as the Desperados. Access to specialist
climbing equipment was at a premium, but this did not prevent
youthful enthusiasm from prevailing.

By the time I met Sam in 1978, he had already acquired formidable experience as a mountaineer. I encountered him in the
Aragon bar on Byres Road, where he was standing in animated
conversation, pint in hand, with a group that included, among
others, Sandy Reid. Sam's passion for climbing, obvious intelligence, sharp wit, and strong dislike and intolerance of conceit and

stuffiness all resonated strongly with me, and so began a long and treasured friendship, a major part of which involved climbing.

I was already an experienced rock climber, but had no experience of snow and ice climbing. When winter arrived, however, I accompanied Sam and Sandy on frequent weekend trips north. They had by now each acquired state-of-the-art winter climbing equipment, including a pair of MacInnes all metal ice-axes with inclined picks. The latter, when employed with rigid 12-point crampons, enabled ice routes to be tackled by the revolutionary technique of 'front-pointing'. I equipped myself similarly and gradually, under the expert guidance of Sam and Sandy, acquired increasing experience in the art of winter climbing. Because of the rapidly changing and unpredictable winter weather in the Scottish mountains, this was not always as straightforward as I had imagined. Frequently, after a long walk to the start of a proposed winter climb, the route was judged to be in poor condition and hence not climbable. The reasons for designating a route to be in poor condition, I learned, were multiple – too much snow, not enough snow, or the wrong type of snow.

The act of climbing usually involves intense physical activity and concentration, but the actual climbing time was far exceeded by time spent travelling, resting, and waiting for good weather to arrive. This provided considerable opportunity for discussion and debate. Sam had strong views on most issues, and heated discussions on philosophy, literature and politics were the norm. The discussions, while passionate and sometimes serious, were interlaced with much hilarity, frequently triggered by comments from Sam. Sandy and I were often the accepting subjects of Sam's sharp wit, but it was not a unidirectional exchange.

Throughout my induction into Scottish climbing, Sam and Sandy were gracious and generous in imparting advice on how to survive in the hostile winter environment. Whether we actually undertook a planned climb was not, it turned out, so important.

What really mattered was journeying into the magnificent Scottish mountains in anticipation of adventure. Invariably the drive back south included a stop-off at the Drovers Inn at Inverarnan for refreshment. As an aside, the Drovers Inn became, in later years, a common venue for the annual hill-walking weekend that Sam organised, primarily for his colleagues at the Southern General Hospital, although I and many others also took great pleasure in attending those memorable events.

The Scottish mountains are not high by European standards, but their latitude, isolation and exposure to gale-force winds and high rainfall make them a serious proposition, especially in winter. The immense rock walls of Ben Nevis and Glen Coe possess a savage grandeur that is without equal in the UK. The high plateaux of the Cairngorms provide a less dramatic but equally challenging climbing ground in a remote and beautiful mountain landscape. Sam climbed extensively in all of these mountainous regions: frequent trips were made to Ben Nevis, Glencoe, and the Cairngorms, as well as to the less accessible Northern Highlands and the Western Isles. Together with Sandy he completed winter traverses of all the great Scottish mountain ridges, including Liathach and An Teallach in the remote Torridon mountains and the Aonach Eagach ridge on the north side of Glencoe – considered by many to be the finest ridge on the British mainland.

Although Sam's first love was the Scottish mountains, he and Sandy climbed much further afield. On several occasions they journeyed to the Alps, usually basing themselves in Chamonix. Their ascents included Mont Blanc and a long list of other routes in the Aiguilles. They also travelled to Zermatt from where they scaled the Matterhorn via the Hornli ridge. This particular ascent had not been without incident: throughout the climb they had encountered queues of climbers competing for access to the route and had to dodge rocks dislodged by climbers that rained on those below like lethal missiles. Fortunately they emerged tired but unharmed. As well as the Alps, Sam and Sandy also climbed in the Atlas Mountains of Morocco – a trip marred by severe gastroenteritis that left them too weak to climb. They also in later years visited the greatest of all mountain ranges, the Himalayas, where they experienced the exhilaration of high-altitude climbing but also the dangers.

While Sam taught me much about winter climbing, I retained the upper hand when it came to pure rock climbing and had, on one particular occasion in 1979, the chance to observe Sam at the limit of his technical rock-climbing ability. The setting was a challenging rock climb several hundred feet long on the Trilleachan Slabs in Glen Etive. This huge sweep of unbroken granite is inclined at 40 degrees, but feels considerably steeper. It provides a thrilling and technically demanding type of climbing where careful balance enables the climber to pad up the rock face and where confidence, rather than physical strength, is the key to success.

Our route on the great central slab ascended directly upwards for over two hundred feet to a long horizontal traverse left along a large overlap, before continuing vertically up again. After a couple of relatively straightforward pitches, Sam was belayed securely to the rock, just below the overlap. I set off, first pulling my way up and onto the upper slab and then delicately moving crab-wise leftwards along its lower edge, following a thin horizontal crack. Eventually I reached a secure belay that signalled the end of the traverse and, with some relief, secured myself to the rock face. In most situations the climber going second is secure in the assumption that, should they fall, the climbing rope will quickly arrest their descent. This pitch was, however, an exception to this rule – Sam, should he fall, faced the unwelcome prospect of a massive pendulum swing across the abrasive lower slab. Secure in the knowledge that I was attached

so securely to the rock and with growing interest in what was
to come, I signalled for Sam to start the long traverse leftwards.
It was, understandably, a nerve-racking experience for him as
he gained the upper slab and calculated the implications of a
slip. After a brief pause he began climbing, slowly at first and
then increasingly fast. To my amusement his legs, by the time he
approached me, were trembling involuntarily. Sam was clearly
very relieved when he completed the traverse, but after a brief
pause the rest of the climb proceeded without incident.

As for Point Five Gully, on that memorable day in 1979,
Sam and I went on to complete our ascent successfully. Having
negotiated the technically challenging lower section on perfect
ice, there came the realisation that we would reach the summit
intact and we both felt elated. For my part, I was glad that I had
accompanied Sam on a route that has a special place in climbing
history and I think he had not, until then, really thought he
would ever complete the climb. On reaching the summit plateau
we basked briefly in the spring sunshine and then traversed the
narrow arête towards Carn Mor Dearg before descending back
to the CIC hut.

We never climbed again at such a high level of technical difficulty in Scotland, but we did complete many other notable
winter routes on Ben Nevis. We even climbed from the luxury
of a hotel on one occasion. The route was Italian Climb – a fine
ice climb, notorious for its susceptibility to potentially fatal slab
avalanches. This risk was uppermost in our minds as we made
the ascent in the warmth of late spring, but fortunately the climb
was without incident and we returned to our hotel in the early
evening suffering from nothing more serious than dehydration.
In what was an amusing coincidence the hotel had organised
a themed 'Italian Evening' and we made the great mistake of
slaking our thirst with large quantities of Chianti. The following
morning we felt, as Sam would say, 'terrible'.

I hope these anecdotes provide some insight into Sam Galbraith, mountaineer and climber. For Sam, as for Sandy and me, serious rock and ice climbing was increasingly eclipsed by hill-walking and skiing trips – less dangerous (mostly) but equally enjoyable mountain activities. Nicola had, under Sam's guidance, become very good at climbing but her real forte was skiing, in which she displayed a grace and poise that Sam could never hope to emulate. New Year holidays in the Cairngorms in the company of Senga and Harry Burns, along with Jean and David Hamilton, were a much anticipated and regular highlight.

While Sam excelled in the urban environment, reaching the top of both the medical and political worlds, the Scottish mountains always held a very special place in his heart. Climbing with Sam gave those of us lucky enough to accompany him a privileged insight into his remarkable character. The exuberance, decisiveness and unwavering confidence displayed in his professional life were apparent, but so too was a sensitivity and vulnerability. There was also humility, but above all a deep humanity. Sam was an inspirational figure and much loved friend. As Dr Wil Rose noted, 'Success is not counted by how high you have climbed but how many people you brought with you.'

Andrew Bradley

Lecturer, Consultant, Professor in Surgery, Western Infirmary, and University of Glasgow, 1978–97; Professor of Surgery, University of Cambridge, 1997 continuing.

II

Philosophers in 'The Aragon'

Harry Burns

Even the combination of great intellect, sharp debating ability, wit and humour in addition to his professional achievements does not explain who Sam was and what he meant to his friends. Sam was one of the kindest, most generous people I ever met. The fact that he tried to hide this aspect of his character behind a gruff and grumpy façade just made him all the more endearing to those of us who made the effort to get to know him.

I first met him in 1975 when I started work in Sir Andrew Kay's Unit as a junior researcher. Our first meeting occurred where so many encounters took place, in the Aragon, a pub in Byres Road, close to the Western Infirmary.

Our first encounter might have turned out badly. Here was I, a private-school boy, educated by Jesuits, while Sam was an atheist from an evangelical Protestant family who took his working-class roots very seriously. On the face of it and given the usual West of Scotland nonsense about religion, things might have gone very badly.

In fact, we got on like a house on fire. Sam began the encounter in the manner I came to know well. 'What school did you go to?' He continued with a series of insults. But he was easy to read. The twinkle in his eyes as he made his standard jibes about posh schools told me this was a test. If I got offended, that told him something about me. I gave as good as I got, and with the same good humour. I had passed the test. After work on a Friday many of us would walk over to the pub for some post-work recreation. The Department of Surgery was always well represented. Many things were discussed.

Friday nights in the Aragon were usually in two parts. We would drift across from the Western Infirmary around 5.30 to discuss the week's work. The married ones, who might live in the suburbs, would usually have one drink and head home, while those of us who were single and lived within walking distance would stay longer. After two or three pints, the discussions would move beyond the limits of work and head for more imaginative areas. Politics, economics, international affairs would be considered and usually dealt with quickly, but often discussion settled on philosophy. Sam was interested in the philosophical basis of his political ideas.

Scottish philosophers were frequently discussed. David Hume, being anti-religion, was a favourite of Sam's. John Rawls and his *Theory of Justice* made it into the Aragon on Fridays, but it was Wittgenstein who had the greatest impact on the customers of the pub.

Ludwig Wittgenstein was an Austrian philosopher who was interested in how the language we use determines how we experience the world. Sandy Reid was quite taken with this idea, but Sam was a bit more sceptical.

This argument was taking place near the door of the pub and new customers were passing by as the debate got more heated. Eventually, in an attempt to underline the absurdity of Sandy's argument, Sam asked: 'If we called this beer glass an elephant, would that mean it would become an elephant?' Not to be outdone, Sandy began a defence of Wittgenstein and the possibility of the 'elephantness' of beer glasses was hotly debated for half an hour. Eventually, one of our group headed through the bar to the toilet. When he came back he was smiling broadly. 'The whole bar is discussing beer glasses and elephants!' Sure enough, in a Glasgow pub on a Friday night, Sam and Sandy had turned everyone's conversation to the thinking of one of the twentieth century's greatest philosophers.

After that argument, it was decided we didn't know enough about Wittgenstein and several of us signed up for an evening class at Glasgow University on Hume and Wittgenstein, led by the head of the Philosophy Department, Ephraim Borowski. Inevitably, those classes ended with us all, Ephraim included, in the Aragon, carrying on the debate.

Sam was an experienced mountaineer and climber, but was always a bit disdainful about skiers, or 'plankers' as he liked to call them. I was a skier! I had done a bit of climbing but was not nearly as accomplished as Sam. On our trips to winter cottages in the Cairngorms, Sam and Sandy would head off climbing while I would usually head for the Coire Cas ski lifts. Eventually, arguments that a really accomplished mountain man needed to be comfortable with skis as well as an ice axe won Sam over. These arguments were helped by the publication of Myrtle Simpson's book on the history of Scottish skiing. This book described skiing as something that had been happening in Scotland since the late nineteenth century, making it legitimate in Sam's eyes. It wasn't just a pursuit for soft toffs while the hard men fought their way up icy gullies.

As a lover of mountains, learning to ski was a new way for Sam to get around them quickly. We enjoyed several continental holidays, usually in a catered chalet. Sam was warned before arrival not to be rude to the chalet girls if they turned out, as they usually did, to be from parts of London close to Sloane Square and had attended fancy Swiss finishing schools. Skiing must have mellowed him, because he was usually well-behaved. If he showed signs of circling to attack, David Hamilton was quick to spot the signs and calm him down.

One particular trip taught him a lesson. We were headed for Verbier in Switzerland. We met at Glasgow Airport at the agreed time for the flight to Geneva. At least, we all did except Sam. He was nowhere to be seen. After we had been hanging about waiting for him, the departure time was approaching when Sam breezed into the airport. He announced that, as a seasoned international traveller, he knew better than to wait in queues. Off he went to the check-in desk only to be told that the flight was now closed and he had missed it! He had to wait for several hours to catch the next flight and was the butt of much abuse when he finally arrived in Switzerland.

If the weekend usually started in the Aragon, almost always it would end with a gathering in the Ashoka in Dumbarton Road. If some had been on call and in Glasgow, usually others had been in the hills. Those who were free would meet on Sunday evening for a curry and to tell tales of the weekend's activities. The Ashoka was the first restaurant in what became a large chain of Indian restaurants in West Central Scotland. It was started by Balbir who became, and still is, a friend. Over the years we met and enjoyed beer and curry in many of Balbir's establishments. The last time I saw Sam was in Balbir's restaurant just a few weeks before he died.

Balbir remembers Sam with great affection. He particularly remembers getting a telling-off from him in the early days of his business. Sam was leaving the restaurant just before it closed. Balbir and his waiters were sitting at a table, having a drink before tidying up for the night. Sam gave them a lecture about the evils of alcohol. The irony was not lost on them!

As a well-known brain surgeon, newly elected MP and bachelor, Sam was seen by some in the media to be something of a catch. One newspaper even listed him as one of Scotland's most eligible bachelors. That suggestion gave his friends plenty of opportunity to get back at him for the abuse we had suffered over the years. The fact was, we knew that, in Nicola, Sam had found the love of his life. It wasn't a matter of who he would marry; it was simply a matter of when.

In the summer of 1987, Sam told me he and Nicola planned to get married and he asked if my wife and I would be witnesses. Of course we would! We were honoured to be asked, but we realised we were probably the only two friends he could trust to keep quiet about it. The plan was to keep the wedding date secret so there would be no press interest. The wedding was arranged for the Kingussie Registry Office. The rule was that a notice of forthcoming weddings had to be posted outside in the three weeks before the planned date. We realised this might have given the game away, and half an hour before it was due, I walked along Ruthven Road to make sure there was no one lurking outside the Office. The coast was clear and the wedding was duly completed with the only guest being our eight-month-old daughter, who kept up a commentary of gurgles throughout the ceremony.

Later that day, friends arrived at Sam's Kingussie house for a party. I think, by then, most had worked out what was going on and we had a memorable evening with two wonderful people.

Sam had an impact on everyone he met. His effect on me and my career was considerable. As a junior surgeon, my duties in the Western Infirmary were to provide initial care for surgical emergencies, including patients with head injuries. I didn't find the training in care of these patients particularly helpful so I asked Sam for a quick tutorial. In the space of an hour, he taught me everything I needed to know about these patients. He was an outstanding teacher.

By 1989, I had been a consultant surgeon for five years. I had spent those years working in the Royal Infirmary in Glasgow where the patients were suffering from many of the illnesses of poverty. I wanted to do something more for them than operate on them. Sam was the obvious person from whom to seek advice. We had spent New Year with Sam and Nicola in Kingussie. One afternoon, I told him about my restlessness. We quickly established that I had no interest in becoming a politician. 'Why don't you go and do community medicine? You could do a lot for poor neighbourhoods from that specialty.' It had never occurred to me to pursue such a career change. I thought about it for about 30 seconds and realised it was the most sensible option available. Sam was like that. He went straight to the heart of the matter with clear thinking and straight talking. The decision was made. It was the best career move I ever made and I owe it to Sam.

Sam and I sparred over many years about religion and the existence of God. Eventually we dropped the subject because we saw we weren't going to change each other's minds. Our last conversation on the matter came after he and Nicola had been at my daughter's wedding in 2012. With good humour he sat through an hour-long Catholic service. He was quite relaxed about the experience and asked a few questions. As I started to respond to some of his questions, he waved me away and said: 'It's OK, Harry, I know you don't believe any of that stuff, anyway.' In saying that, he was, I suppose, paying me a compliment.

The closest I ever got Sam to acknowledging that the existence of God might be possible was on a weekend up at the cottage we rented near Feshiebridge. Our usual vigorous debate ended with Sam concluding that the probability that a god existed was about the same as the probability of us eventually finding a toilet roll in orbit around the planet Jupiter.

'That's a small probability, Sam, but it's not a zero probability,' I said.

His response was: 'No, it's non-zero, but it's infinitesimally small, so why would you live your life based on such a small probability?'

'Sam, no matter how small it is, so long as the possibility exists, why would you NOT live your life based on it?'

That was the last significant debate we had on the possibility of a god. It made me feel better after his death. Sam, and his friend Sandy, were generous, caring and compassionate. I have no doubt that, if an afterlife exists, they were welcomed in. I imagine them both, sitting in the heavenly equivalent of the Aragon, Sam insulting passing angels about their weight, and both discussing which mountain they will head for next.

Rest in peace, guys!

Professor Sir Harry Burns

Surgical Trainee and Consultant Surgeon, Western Infirmary and Royal Infirmary, Glasgow, 1975–89; Chief Medical Officer for Scotland, 2005–14.

12

Education, Ethics and the Politics of Health

Robin Downie

Many commentators and obituary writers stressed that Sam was not a 'professional politician', meaning that he had a 'hinterland' – his very successful career as a neurosurgeon. This of course is correct and was important in the shaping of his career and personality. But there was more than one hinterland: it is also well known that he was a skilled and experienced mountaineer, and of course a devoted husband and father. I got to know him in yet another context where his views on medical education, health and politics began to be shaped. This was at the meetings of the Glasgow Medical Group (GMG).

The term 'medical group' nowadays refers mainly to GP practices and what they can offer. The internet provides information on medical groups of this kind. Sam would not have objected to that. But nowadays the term also refers to private practices offering services such as cosmetic surgery, and sometimes providing prices for what is on offer. The information on these is usually accompanied by pictures of smiling doctors and nurses and testimonials from satisfied patients. Not Sam's sort of thing at all! But the GMG of the 1970s and '80s was something quite different. It consisted of students and staff from assorted disciplines, medical and non-medical, and we met every couple of weeks to talk about medicine and the NHS from many different points of view. There were similar medical groups of this kind attached to most medical schools. Sam was a strong supporter of them and frequently took part in the discussions. It was through these meetings that I was privileged to meet him.

It may be of interest to say something about the history of medical groups, why they came into existence and why Sam strongly approved of them. One important reason was the desire – expressed by students as well as some staff – to have some discussion of ethical issues. It is true that what was called 'medical ethics' was taught at Glasgow and in other medical schools during this early period (up to 1970), but it is easy to forget what this consisted of and how far removed it was from what would now be considered medical ethics, or health-care ethics or bioethics (to introduce the range of terms now in use). What was taught before 1970 consisted mainly of etiquette – precedence in the ward rounds for example – and instruction on how to behave in court, and how to avoid being sued. It was assumed that anything else would be acquired by osmosis from senior consultants on the ward round. Training in communication skills did not exist as a separate component in the curriculum, and as far as patients were concerned paternalism reigned supreme. This emphasis on what was considered medical professionalism meant that anyone who was not medically qualified was not regarded as worth listening to. There was some unease about this situation, however, and the unease led to the rise of 'medical groups'. These consisted of staff and students from other university departments, such as sociology, politics, moral philosophy and law. Contributions from these varied perspectives broadened the idea of medical professionalism, and medical groups can be seen as acting as a kind of transition between the early days of ethics as etiquette and doing as the consultant did, and the full-blown teaching of medical ethics with student involvement as an essential part of the curriculum, as is common nowadays.

Sam approved of the establishment of medical groups such as the GMG, because he saw them as providing the broader educational dimension which many felt was lacking in the training of doctors at that time. He contributed to this educational dimension, and the discussions in turn helped to shape his political views on medical education, the NHS and wider issues.

Sam was able to make successful contributions partly because he had what can be called 'street cred'. Medical students are a confident bunch and do not always take seriously points of view other than received medical opinion delivered by medical consultants. But when a neurosurgeon speaks then he will certainly be listened to, and what he says will be thought about. For example, it is common for medical students to interpret the problems of life in medical terms and to look for medical solutions. But when Sam told them that many health problems, perhaps the majority, are caused by lifestyle and diet, and that lifestyle and diet are themselves partly or mainly the result of poverty, then they listened. Indeed, speaking more generally, I think it correct to say that Sam's major contribution to politics was to convince ministers of the link between poverty and ill health. Of course, this had been known before. For example, the well-researched Black Report (cynically published on the August Bank Holiday of 1980) made this clear, but when the points are stressed by a neurosurgeon then they are taken seriously.

Sam could also bring clarity to the discussions. I remember one discussion on smoking (and of course we are talking about the late 1970s or early 1980s). The lecturer argued for a ban on the grounds that it would save a lot of money. Sam pointed out in discussion that a ban on smoking would mean that people would live longer and that this would cost the government in the end more by way of a drain on pensions. His argument was that the only reason for a ban on smoking was a health reason.

Some commentators have suggested that Sam did not suffer fools gladly, hinting that he had a touch of the arrogance which (fairly or not) is often said to be a characteristic of surgeons. Certainly, Tam Dalyell (I think) reported a conversation in which Sam said, 'Surgeons are always decisive people, the sort of guys who walk right down the centre of a corridor, while physicians walk along the side.' No doubt decisiveness is a necessary quality for a surgeon, but I never found him arrogant in discussion. He would listen politely to student views and was on the whole soft-spoken. Not always though. Once we had a talk from a well-known QC – another walker-down-the-centre-of-corridors – and Sam strongly disagreed with him. The rest of us were under the seats!

If Sam contributed to these meetings of the GMG he also gained from them. He would listen carefully to the contributions from students and staff from other university departments. Contributions from these quarters gave him a wider perspective than that of the purely medical, or at least helped him develop an existing turn of mind. It must be remembered that medical education has changed a great deal since Sam's day, and that he would have emerged from a training which was narrow and highly focused, and perhaps not entirely patient-friendly. But lawyers – such as Ian Kennedy, and in Glasgow Professor Sheila McLean – were arguing forcefully at that time for the patient's right to know. Discussions with the lawyers certainly affected Sam's views on medical education, although it was only after his own experiences as a patient that he said he fully understood what patients are put through.

This period of transition from the early days of medical training to the inclusion of medical ethics as an essential part of the medical curriculum was not without its problems. I remember being approached by the Dean at the time to enquire whether I would be willing to do some teaching with the undergraduates on ethical issues. But I was immediately telephoned by the Professor of Forensic Medicine, who said in no uncertain terms: 'I want you to be clear, Downie, that I teach ethics in this university.' Fortunately, I was able to team up with Ken Calman and we developed a successful double act, teaching a wide range of ethical and communication issues, and involving the students in group discussion. Other distinguished consultants with an interest in ethics also got involved in raising difficult issues in specialised areas. For example, Callum Macnaughton discussed the ethical problems concerned with *in vitro* fertilisation, and Bryan Jennett discussed brain-stem death. Sam was pleased with all that, but I reckon he would have been even more pleased with the introduction of medical humanities – which enables students to take as part of their curriculum some non-medical subject. I remember running a special study module on Plato's *Republic* with about a dozen medical students. The students had just finished their family placements and were full of the importance of the family. But Plato rubbishes the family! The clash of ideas reminded me of the discussions in the GMG that Sam enjoyed, and he would certainly have approved of the new possibilities in medical education.

The exchange of ideas with staff and students with other approaches to life enabled Sam to develop his early political ideas into his full-blown political philosophy. It was as if his critique of medical education laid the foundation for his critique of Scottish education and indeed of Scottish society more generally. Although he was Scottish to the core he was nevertheless able to distance himself and see the many weaknesses and contradictions in Scottish society, such as the ability to combine the cringe factor with the boastfulness of 'Here's tae us, wha's like us.' In the preface to Carol Craig's excellent book *The Scots' Loss of Confidence*, Kirsty Wark tells the story of a conversation in a Greenock pub (Sam's home town, of course). Someone was proudly boasting of a local lad who had made good. But his story was capped by someone else who said, 'Aye, but his uncle was an alcoholic.' Sam would have appreciated both the humour and the truth in that very plausible anecdote. It distils much of what he wanted to correct in Scottish society.

Many of the GMG meetings were held in the Western Infirmary in Glasgow and Sam often managed to organise sandwiches, at least for the speakers. I don't know where they came from. They were certainly not from a drug company – Sam would have choked on a sandwich from a drug company. No doubt he used his undoubted charm on the catering staff. As often as not there were sandwiches left, and I can remember him scooping them up into his briefcase and saying: 'I like a sangwidge [sic] for my tea.' This of course was before the days of Nicola!

In these early days before his political career really got going he was not only developing his skills as a neurosurgeon but also becoming aware of much wider issues and their complexities, and the many different possible approaches to them. It was Mark Twain (I think) who said: 'If your only tool is a hammer, all your problems become nails!' But not all problems are nails, and Sam realised that, both in medical education and in politics more generally, a variety of tools is necessary.

Robin Downie

Professor of Moral Philosophy, 1969–2002; Emeritus Professor 2002 continuing, University of Glasgow.

13

Grounded in the Good of the People

Harpreet Kohli

It was a warm Saturday morning in summer at Ross Priory. The game we were playing looked like a fair approximation of golf and we were enjoying it. However, that was not what was on my mind. Looking down from the third tee to the fairway and beyond to Loch Lomond, Ben Lomond and the Cobbler on the horizon, the realisation dawned on me. From what Sam had just said, I had met him, without being aware of it, long before I got to know him. Ray and Stewart, our partners on the round (and by far the better golfers), were a little bemused, as Sam and I spent the rest of the round reminiscing – and slicing our drives.

I had met Sam in the Ashoka Restaurant (now called the Ashoka Westend) in Argyle Street, close to Glasgow University, when, as a teenager in the mid-1970s, I worked there as a barman and waiter. I have the recollection of a group of, in the main, polite men who frequented the Ashoka, but whose language was colourful. To an 18-year-old they looked old – at least 25 years of age – and I never really got chatting to them because, well, they were old and I had my teenager things to do. So without knowing it, I had served Sam and his friends pints of Tuborg lager and the Ashoka curries which were at that time becoming renowned throughout Glasgow.

It was only when I left Glasgow to study (and do my penance) in Edinburgh, that I heard of Sam and his activities. As a medical student in Edinburgh in the late 1970s, I was far removed from the world of medical politics but I became aware of this young neurosurgeon in Glasgow who was becoming active in politics. I learnt also of Sam's flirtation with the breakaway Scottish Labour Party (SLP) which Jim Sillars was instrumental in setting up. The SLP imploded because of entryism by the International Marxist Group (IMG, which was 'the British Section of the Fourth International'). It was with much pleasure that Sam later recounted his expulsion from the SLP as an entryist (although he had no connections with the IMG) and the fact that he learned of this as he lay on a beach in Texas.

I cannot imagine how anyone would think that Sam could have been in the IMG. For those who remember the 1970s, there was a plethora of leftist groups, each one more ideologically pure than the next. Names such as the Internationalist Socialists, the Revolutionary Socialist League (also known as the Militant Tendency which was 'not a party, just discussion groups of like-minded individuals'), the Revolutionary Communist Group, the Revolutionary Communist Tendency, and the IMG will bring a nostalgic tear to the eye of student and extra-parliamentary left-wing politicians of that era.

The navel-gazing of the left didn't help when Thatcher came to power in the 1979 UK general election. What followed was a Conservative government which attacked the rights of workers and the social wage, ripped the heart out of many communities throughout the UK and exacerbated inequalities in Britain. As a medical student, I became a member of the Medical Practitioners' Union (MPU) which was for doctors and medical students who did not wish to join the BMA and wanted to resist Thatcher's policies against the NHS. The MPU was more radical than the BMA and it also had links to the trade union movement and the Labour Party. The MPU was founded in 1914 as the Medico-Political Union, becoming the MPU in 1922. By the 1970s it was part of the Association of Scientific, Technical and Managerial Staffs (ASTMS) trade union and since then it has been part of various trade unions – the Manufacturing, Science and Finance (MSF), Amicus and, currently, Unite.

I was, by now, following Sam's developing career in the MPU and also the Labour Party, but it was only after I graduated in 1981 and became a junior doctor that I finally met Sam (again). The occasion was a meeting of the South East Scotland Branch of the MPU. There were about 10 of us who met in a member's house in west Edinburgh and Sam had been invited to come and speak. At that time the SE Scotland MPU was worried about the expansion of private medical practice in Edinburgh and was looking at ways of countering this. My impressions of the meeting are from memory because no notes survive, but three things struck me as I listened to Sam. First, despite his increasingly high profile, he was very down to earth and easy to talk to – unlike the neurosurgeons I encountered as a medical student and a junior doctor! Second, he was very helpful to the branch in undertaking actions which were realistic and achievable. Instead of waiting for a revolution that was beyond the horizon, there were things which we could do now. Third, it legitimised the view we, as MPU members, had of the NHS by having the support and interest of a high-profile politically aware doctor. It was also during this period that Sam, together with some like-minded consultants, donated their salary rise from the Conservative government to patients at the hospital in Lochgilphead. The money, I understand, was used to buy a boat and improved the health and wellbeing of the patients to no small extent.

When I moved to Glasgow in 1985 I met Sam more frequently at the meetings of the West of Scotland Branch of the MPU – and in the Halt bar after meetings. I can clearly remember him giving me advice, over a pint, on becoming a parent, the night before I became a father for the first time. I had only the one pint to allow me to drive Kate, if required, to the Queen Mother's Hospital for the delivery, but fortunately Siobhan decided to wait until the next day before coming into the world. Sam used the occasion to offer me expansive advice on children and how to raise them. Only later did I wonder what sort of advice Sam was dishing out in the absence of any practical experience himself at that point!

Sam's view of his developing political activities was that they were a natural extension of his work as a doctor. There is no doubt that in the 1970s and 1980s he was exploring what contribution he could make for the greater good of society. He obviously felt that as a leading neurosurgeon in Glasgow he hadn't contributed nearly enough to society. I also think that, as an emerging activist and politician, Sam was firmly grounded in the commonweal of people that he was born into, grew up in and served. Sam recognised the opportunities that he got to go beyond the working-class environment of Greenock and which allowed him to go to Glasgow University to study medicine. But he also recognised that other, equally talented, children did not get a chance to develop their full potential.

As a doctor he was fiercely protective of an NHS based on people's health needs, not whether they could pay for the treatment. It was no surprise that he became the President of the MPU. This also paved the way for him to become a Labour MP in the UK Parliament in 1987. He was, of course, one of those rare beasts among British and Scottish politicians – someone who made his name in the real world of work and then became a politician. In 1997 when he became Minister for Health in Scotland, many credited him with making the links between poverty, ill health and health inequalities politically acceptable to discuss and act upon, after 18 years of Conservative government which had denied these links. They were the original poverty- and inequality-deniers.

Sam's life experiences undoubtedly contributed to his perspectives as a politician, including having responsibility as

Minister for Health in Scotland. He had experience of the NHS at all levels – of primary care and general practice, of his local hospitals such as the Western Infirmary and Gartnavel General, and of the specialist care at the Freeman Hospital transplant centre in Newcastle. He also understood the NHS intimately in his roles as a patient, a parent, the partner of a health care worker, and a doctor. He appreciated patients' perspectives and as a consultant he practised patient-centred care. His ill health and subsequent lung transplant gave him further insight into just how much doctors and health staff put patients through. His philosophy with patients was that you should 'always try to do the right thing for your patient, not what the patient wants'. Of course, it was good if both these perspectives were aligned. Translated into politics, for Sam this philosophy meant 'always try to do the right thing, not the most popular or politically convenient thing to do'. I suspect this approach came as a shock to many in Westminster and Holyrood.

Although these reflections are primarily about Sam's emergence as an activist and a politician, it was when I got to know Sam and Nicola as friends that I could place my contacts with Sam in the MPU and the Labour Party at that time in context. I only fully appreciated this latterly with Sam over the cups of tea, or an occasional malt, when chatting (and with me sweating) in the sauna-like temperatures in his house. Who knew my journey with Sam, which had started with serving him curries in the Ashoka, would end here?

Harpreet Kohli

Trainee and Consultant in Public Health Medicine, Glasgow and Lanarkshire, 1985–2008; Director of Public Health, Lanarkshire, 2008 continuing.

14

Turning Bearsden Red

Grahame Smith

I hardly knew Sam when he walked into my office at the STUC's headquarters in Woodlands Terrace in Glasgow to ask me to run his 1987 election campaign. His request came just a few weeks before the election was due to be called. It followed a period of turmoil and infighting within Strathkelvin Constituency Labour Party (CLP), something that seems to be a Party speciality, over his continuation as Labour's candidate, which had culminated in the resignation of the original choice as election agent, Strathclyde Regional Councillor Tom Rae.

Unbeknown to all but his family, closest friends, the Labour hierarchy and the Constituency Party officers, Sam was ill and would subsequently be diagnosed with the lung condition fibrosing alveolitis. Shortly before local Party members were informed and Sam's continued candidacy confirmed, I was told of his illness, in confidence, by Brian Wilson, his close friend and at the time the Labour candidate in Cunninghame North. He also sounded me out about taking on the role of election agent.

I was not an obvious choice. I had never run an election campaign. I had never had a proper conversation with Sam and was a member of one of the few local branches, the Auchinairn branch, not to nominate him as Labour's candidate. Although his politics did not align with those of most branch activists, a split in votes for the other candidates resulted in a nomination for Danny Carrigan, an official of the Engineering, Electrical,

Telecommunications and Plumbing Union (EETPU), a union firmly on the right wing of the Party. In the mind of some CLP members, I and other branch delegates were clearly 'not supporters of Sam'.

I didn't vote for Sam at the branch nominating meeting, principally because he didn't attend to present his case. He was mountaineering in the Himalayas at the time! My vote went to Iain MacDonald, a Regional Councillor from the centre-left of the Party. Of course, while I didn't know Sam, I knew of him through his involvement in the Medical Practitioners' section of the STUC-affiliated union, the Association of Scientific, Technical and Managerial Staffs (ASTMS) and by dint of his many platform appearances at anti-NHS privatisation rallies and other campaigning events.

I did vote for him at the final constituency selection meeting at which he defeated, amongst others, Anne McGuire, who was to become the Labour MP for Stirling at the 1997 election, defeating arch-Thatcherite Michael Forsyth. While Sam won the selection comfortably, some held reservations about his candidacy. He carried some political baggage from his association with Jim Sillars' Scottish Labour Party, some thought his politics were a little too far to the left and some railed against selecting a candidate just to appeal to the suburban middle class. Others believed, with some justification, that he could best serve the interests of humanity and indeed the interests of the Labour Party through continuing to practise as a world-leading neurosurgeon, and through the impact that a high-profile health professional such as he had when speaking out against the Tories' NHS privatisation agenda.

I agreed to take on the election agent role. To allay any concerns within the CLP about my suitability, I was to work alongside Ben Smith, former Scottish Secretary of the public services union NALGO, a former member of the Communist

Party, and someone who exerted significant influence over the internal politics of Strathkelvin CLP.

I soon discovered that there had been very little planning or preparation undertaken for the impending campaign, save for the purchase of the thousands of envelopes needed for the one free mailshot available to each candidate.

From the outset, Sam was completely open with me about his medical condition and insistent that it should never interfere with how I wanted to run the campaign or the demands I should make on him as a candidate.

Strathkelvin and Bearsden was a new parliamentary constituency first contested at the 1983 general election. Lying outside the Glasgow city boundary to the north, it had little coherence as a constituency, appearing to have been formed from what was left after changes had been made to the boundaries of surrounding constituencies. It was geographically and culturally diffuse. It included Bearsden in the west, one of the most affluent areas of Scotland; the rural areas of Lennoxtown and Torrance, whose gravitational pull was towards Stirlingshire; the Glasgow suburbs of Bishopbriggs and Lenzie; and in the east, the ancient and somewhat parochial town of Kirkintilloch.

When first contested in 1983, the seat was won by a prominent Conservative, Michael Hirst, with a majority of 3,700 over the Liberal Democrats. Labour came third, a further 1,500 votes behind, the consequence of a disastrous national campaign and a discordant local Party.

Although it was one of the Party's target seats at the 1987 election, principally because Sam was the candidate, some in Keir Hardie House, the Party's Scottish headquarters, saw little prospect of success. Jimmy Allison, the Party's legendary Scottish organiser, while generous with his advice to a novice election agent, told me in no uncertain terms that we had no chance of winning.

We ran the campaign as if it were a by-election and Sam won with a majority of 2,452 over Hirst. It was a victory that had little to do with my capabilities as an agent. It had much more to do with Sam's appeal as a candidate and the commitment and dedication of local Party workers and those who came from neighbouring safe seats in Glasgow to lend their support. We were also the recipients of significant union backing.

Andy Cochrane, Eleanor and Joe Di Paola, David and Hilda Butler, John and Helen Clugston and Ben and Mildred Smith ran the local election rooms, some from their own homes. Tragically, a few weeks into the campaign Ben collapsed and died, which cast a huge shadow over our victory.

A high-profile visit from Labour Party leader Neil Kinnock gave our campaign national publicity. It was memorable not just for the news coverage of his and Sam's kick-about with a group of youngsters at Bishopbriggs Sports Centre but for the near pneumonia inflicted on the children of two Party members we persuaded to stay in the swimming pool for more than two hours in order to pose for a photograph with the late-running leader. While most considered the visit a great success and a major boost to our campaign, I later discovered that some of our Kirkintilloch comrades were aggrieved that the visit hadn't been to their local swimming pool!

Sam's victory was just one of a number of Labour successes in Scotland. The Party took 50 seats, an increase of 9 from 1983, and ousted a number of prominent Tories apart from Hirst, including Michael Ancram and Gerry Malone.

One of the peculiarities of being an election agent is that during a campaign you see very little of your candidate. You arrange the workplace visits, the meetings with community influencers, the targeted canvassing, the photo opportunities, and make sure your candidate is accompanied by someone you are confident can ensure that they are where they should be, that they arrive and depart on time, and avoid dropping a calamitous clanger. In the 1987 campaign the role of Sam's minder was expertly performed by Bob Arnott, an economics professor whose politics sat somewhat to the left of Sam's. Bob regularly reported back to me on his political debates with Sam as he drove him to engagements across the constituency. Although Sam's health was never an issue during the campaign, Bob was under instructions to ensure he had sufficient time to rest and to prepare for his next engagement.

As a campaigner, Sam was at his best when talking to voters face to face. He exuded the sort of self-confidence that comes from operating on someone's brain for hours on end! The bedside manner he employed as a surgeon easily transferred to his political campaigning, although his directness and sense of humour could easily be mistaken for downright rudeness. More than once I was informed by a shocked Party worker of some derogatory remark he had made to a pensioner about her hat or to a parent about how they had dressed their child. This, of course, was quite ironic, given Sam's choice of baggy jumpers and that he often looked as if he had been dragged through a hedge backwards.

In the few candidates' debates that took place he more than held his own with Hirst, a vastly more experienced politician. When Hirst sought to exploit his own anti-abortion stance at a Justice and Peace Rally at St Matthews Church hall in Bishopbriggs, Sam firmly held and cogently argued his pro-choice position and in the end clearly won the debate.

Following his election, Sam offered me the opportunity to run his constituency office. I declined. I had a great job at the STUC and had no appetite to take on a role which might aggravate rather than defuse the simmering in-fighting within the CLP. I believe that Sam made the offer out of a sense of obligation. He would have known that my appointment would not have sat well with his desire to stay well clear of the internal politics of the CLP, something which led ultimately to the end of our candidate-agent relationship.

My suggestion that he ask Hilda Butler to take on the role was without doubt the best piece of advice I ever gave him. Hilda did an exceptional job, not only managing his office but in managing Sam. Unfortunately, the location of his office in Bearsden was yet another issue to exercise the Kirkintilloch comrades.

The success of Sam's 1992 campaign bucked the trend in Scotland. Labour dropped to 49 seats, losing a seat to the Tories, and saw its share of the vote decline by 3.4 per cent. In Strathkelvin and Bearsden, while the Tory vote increased by 2.6 per cent, the Labour vote rose by 4.1 per cent and Sam's majority increased to 3,162. Sam and Nigel Griffiths in Edinburgh South were the only Labour candidates in Scotland to secure an increase in their share of the vote.

Despite continuing friction in the CLP, I continued as Sam's agent for the 1992 campaign. With more time to prepare, with most of the local campaign team still in place and with the opportunity to promote Sam's record as an effective local MP, much of that down to Hilda's effectiveness in running his office, we were confident of retaining the seat. We targeted the Liberal Democrat vote in Bearsden, Bishopbriggs and Lenzie, a strategy which, despite being remarkably successful, was resented by some in other parts of the constituency to which fewer resources were devoted.

I recall it as a long and gruelling campaign with which Sam coped remarkably well, despite still recovering from the lung transplant he had undergone two years earlier. We had tremendous support again from Party members from across the Central Belt and from the unions, and an array of high-profile campaigners came to lend their support.

During a visit from Sam's close friend Donald Dewar, we discovered a past connection between us. In a break from campaigning, I took Sam and Donald to my Mum's for a mug of tea. As they munched their way through her home baking, Sam realised that he had come across her many years before. As a child, although connected to the Elim Pentecostal Church in Greenock, he attended the Sunday School at Orangefield Baptist Church in the town where my father had been the Superintendent. He recalled, almost 40 years later, my Mum as a young woman with a small child; not me, as it turned out, but my older brother.

In 1997, the national swing to Labour made safe what had been a marginal seat when Sam was first elected. He won by a majority of 16,292, with 52.9 per cent of the vote, a 10 per cent increase from 1992.

A demand from the CLP to have Sam be more accountable to the wishes of the local Party resulted in the decision over the appointment of his election agent being taken effectively out of his hands. Having no desire to assert his candidate's prerogative to choose an agent for fear of becoming embroiled in the internal politics of the CLP, Sam relieved me of the agent's responsibilities.

We worked together on occasion after he became the Scottish Office Health Minister and I took on responsibility for health policy at the STUC. He asked me to draft the circular to health boards that ended the privatisation of hospital cleaning and catering services. At a meeting with health unions, I witnessed him demolish erstwhile colleagues from the BMA over their attempts to justify their failure to reduce waiting lists and times. Stretched out on his chair, as was his way, at a 45-degree angle to the floor, with his hands behind his head, he countered every excuse they had to offer. He was very proud that, when a surgeon, he never had a waiting list.

In truth, despite being a former President of the Medical Practitioners' Union, he had little time for trade unions and the STUC in particular. He considered unions to be insufficiently loyal to the Party, expecting them to be cheerleaders rather than critical friends, and viewed them as a barrier to the advancement of the New Labour project that he came to embrace.

Grahame Smith

Sam Galbraith's Election Agent, 1987, 1992; General Secretary, Scottish Trades Union Congress, 2005 continuing.

15

Working for Sam

Hilda Butler

'We'd be lucky to get this person to stand in our constituency. It's a Sam Galbraith . . . It's that Sam Galbraith I saw in George Square one lunchtime, campaigning for the nurses on an open-topped bus.'

David, my husband, had just been meeting a possible parliamentary candidate.

It was *the* Sam Galbraith.

A hospital consultant out campaigning for the nurses? Not usual, but then neither was Sam. He was duly selected to stand and he was a unique candidate.

His first general election campaign in 1987 was extraordinary. Grahame Smith of the STUC was a superb election agent then and again in 1992. He organised a full programme of campaigning events for Sam and was ably assisted by Joe Di Paola of NALGO, the public services union. Grahame and Joe, who always carried a somewhat mysterious black briefcase which impressed the campaigners no end, clearly meant business.

Picture Sam seeing the commuters off at 7 a.m. at the stations in Bearsden, one of the leafier parts of the constituency, with a breezy and confident, 'Good morning! Now I can count on your vote on polling day, can't I?'

Quite often a stunned silence followed, to which Sam would respond with a friendly tap on the shoulder and a cheery, 'Don't worry about it!' But an awful lot of them, who were needed to win the seat, must have voted for him in the end when pencil met ballot paper.

Sam was a leader. He inspired people and they came from all over and from all walks of life to campaign for him in all parts of the constituency. On the eve of the poll there were queues of people wanting to deliver leaflets from him to every household in the constituency.

It was a famous victory. Sam, with the support of Grahame and all his campaign team and the hundreds of people who worked for him (he used to say you can do nothing without 'the troops'), had achieved what not long before had seemed the impossible task of taking a Tory stronghold in a three-way marginal contest. He was elected the Labour MP for Strathkelvin and Bearsden. The title of his maiden speech in the House of Commons on Friday 23 October 1987 was 'Politics is Health'.

A few weeks later our doorbell rang one afternoon. It was Sam and Grahame Smith. I was lying down in bed and descended in my dressing gown, whereupon Sam fell to musing on what Bearsden woman does of an afternoon. That morning I had been diagnosed with breast cancer and was in a state of shock.

It was a complete surprise that Sam had come to offer me the job as his secretary, because he only knew us through the election campaign when we first worked for him as the Bearsden organisers, but he sat me down and told me this diagnosis was, in his words, 'no big deal'. While his medical colleagues, to all of whom we owe everything, took my condition in hand, Sam made interim secretarial arrangements. He and Nicola, his wife, visited and encouraged with more talk of no big deals.

Few people would have allowed the long time necessary for treatment and recovery to someone before they start a job. Sam did and I am even more grateful to him now than I realised then, as I am to Grahame who – as I learned only recently – suggested me for the post.

Sam had his own much bigger deal than mine. He was completely matter-of-fact about it and never complained. He had a single lung transplant, outliving all expectations, and the rest is an amazing history of a life fulfilled in family and work.

On 1 April 1988 Sam's constituency office opened and, with no secretarial staff in London, it covered the constituency and Westminster as well as Holyrood in due course. Wilma McBride, another secretary recruited later, was a meticulous worker and a great asset to Sam's secretariat.

As a Member of Parliament, Sam was committed to helping his constituents and remarkable for the speed with which he responded to problems raised with him in the constituency and at his MP's surgeries. Among these were issues relating to health and education, immigration and asylum seekers, the Benefits Agency, the Child Support Agency, the Law Society of Scotland, and the now defunct Press Complaints Commission.

He would immediately identify the crux of the problem, cut through the red tape and deal with the matter, always letting his constituents know right away the action he was taking on their behalf and keeping them fully informed throughout.

It is fascinating that sometimes issues raised in the constituency highlight anomalies in the law, such as the benefits then payable to people with mesothelioma and other industrial diseases. People with these conditions could receive a lump sum compensation payment and could claim disability benefit.

The first anomaly revealed by a case in Sam's constituency was that the lump sum awarded to someone who had died was almost half the amount made to someone who was still alive. He believed this was wrong because the award was to compensate the family for loss of earnings, and he raised the case of his constituent in the relevant Statutory Instruments Committee in Parliament in March 1993.

The second anomaly highlighted by the constituency case was that the date of the award of benefit was the date of diagnosis by a statutory medical board, and not the date of the medical diagnosis which could have preceded it by some time. Sam wanted the statutory board to have the power to award both compensation and benefit from the date of the medical diagnosis. This was extremely important because the lump sum would then not be diminished if the person had died and the disability benefit would be paid retrospectively from the date of the medical diagnosis.

MPs are lobbied about a wide range of issues from genetically modified crops to animal rights, and they receive large postbags on legislation to be debated in the House of Commons. Sam would carefully consider the concerns raised with him. If his own view differed, he was clear and unequivocal in the responses to his constituents, however unpopular that might be. An example of this was the huge lobby in favour of David Alton's Abortion (Amendment) Bill 1987 which proposed the reduction of the upper time limit for abortion. Sam was against reducing the time limit and explained to his constituents that in his judgement it was a woman's right to choose what to do in consultation with her doctors.

In addition to the surgeries there were constituency visits to schools, hospitals, care homes, leisure centres, community groups and businesses, as well as constituency coffee mornings, lunch clubs, social evenings, open days, fêtes and galas. There were projects to launch and premises to open, like our doctors' surgery extension in Bearsden, where a plaque commemorates the occasion in August 1996.

Driving the MP to these commitments was something which all our family enjoyed doing at one time or other. Sam's directions were always precise, but always just that moment too late, so imagine being told to reverse back up on to one of the famed roundabouts at Cumbernauld when we were further afield and I went wrong. And, worse still, imagine doing it . . . Sam could be very persuasive.

He gave talks on many subjects and once delivered an entire lecture on the outdoors, a subject close to his heart, referring throughout to 'the Royal Society for the Prevention of Birds'. All my eloquent, though necessarily silent, entreaties from the front row were powerless to prevent him from preventing these birds, but the talk was a great success. The talks always were, especially when I had ventured beforehand that he couldn't possibly say what he said he was going to say. He always did. Of course.

There was the task of retrieving his lost property: the coat (somewhere on a train in England – a substantial garment you'd have thought it difficult to lose); the specs (conference organiser to secretary: 'Gold half-moons? I'm bloody sure they were on his nose when he left!'); the pills (flown up by a pilot on a later scheduled flight from London – probably no longer an option).

And there was copious correspondence with memorable letters like the one to Maria Fyfe, the MP for Maryhill. In it he referred to 'the wifies', as he liked to describe the fair sex and as Maria herself recounts in her memories of Sam. Typing the otherwise perfectly serious letter Sam had dictated to her, I felt compelled to put a heartfelt *cri de cœur* in square brackets: '[I can't believe I'm typing this, Maria . . .]' and the letter was duly despatched to her. (Cf orthographic variation: 'wifey'.)

There was the thrill, even in opposition, of Sam being appointed Labour Health Spokesman in 1988, then Employment Spokesman in 1992. And finally government at last, and Labour Minister for Health and the Arts under Donald Dewar at the Scottish Office in London from 1997 to 1999.

Sam greatly admired and valued his civil servants, but I remember one talking to him on the phone and thinking that what he was saying wasn't our health policy. Sam clarified the policy in the continuing call, and having the power to implement Labour policies was tremendous. It was the reason he went into politics: to improve people's lives, especially through policies on health, housing, education and employment.

At that time Labour candidates could stand for both Westminster and the Scottish Parliament, and Sam was elected to both with large majorities (1997 general election, 16,292; 1999 Scottish Parliament election, 12,121). Further ministerial appointments followed at Holyrood, where he was Minister for Children and Education (1999–2000), then Minister for Environment, Sport and Culture (2000–01). The pressure on ministers can be intense.

Sam was a prolific writer for the press and numerous publications on various subjects, especially the NHS, including articles on hospital food, rationing of health care, the internal market in health, health screening and junior doctors' hours. He wrote about being a patient himself and about climbing and the outdoors. He wrote obituaries and reviewed books, and he wrote weekly articles for *Scotland on Sunday* when it was launched.

In his eloquent obituary of W.H. Murray, the great Scottish writer and mountaineer, in the *West Highland Free Press* (April 1996), Sam wrote that Bill Murray was one of his heroes, and with his father and mother, 'was the main force behind my life-long love of the mountains. He introduced me to a paradise from which I shall not depart.'

One of his articles was about the golden rules when talking to patients (*Glasgow Herald*, January 1991) which included never lying to them, but never forcing information on them either; looking them straight in the eye and giving them plenty of time; and never leaving them without hope.

From time to time people would come up to Sam at a talk or meeting, and even in the street when he was out campaigning, to say that he had saved their lives when they were his patients. They had never forgotten him, and he had clearly practised medicine according to his own golden rules.

They were the same golden rules he applied when constituents came to see him at his surgeries or in his office. He had the gift of immediately putting people at their ease, and inspiring confidence in them that he would do his best to help them, as he invariably did.

In the summer of 2014, one of the last times I saw him, we had been talking and agreed that in retirement the ideal was to continue to do some work, but not too much and it had to be real work. That's what he did – though it was much more than a little work – as Chair of the Scottish Maritime Museum Trust, at the General Medical Council and in the Scottish Tribunals Service.

In addition to the great variety of the job in the constituency, working for Sam was also great fun with much merciless leg-pulling, at which he was a past master. But the discussions we had, often when driving him to various places, were one of the best things about working for him. I would arrive in the office after one such discussion the previous day with my irrefutable response ready, secure in the knowledge that I'd got him this time.

'Oh, for heaven's sake [or possibly more colourful words to that effect], Hilda! Has it taken you all night to think of that?' Then, without further ado, he swiftly demolished the irrefutable response.

Sam's outstanding quality was loyalty: loyalty, above everything else, to his family – Nicola, Mhairi, Heather and Fiona, four wonderfully liberated wifies to whom he was devoted, as they were to him; loyalty to his friends and colleagues; and loyalty to his Party.

He was unfailingly loyal to the Labour Party, but he never demanded a blind loyalty from others to political ideas if, like us, they believed Labour was moving too far away from the fundamental principles for which it stood originally. He simply continued the work in hand of trying to show us the error of our ways. It was a continuing discussion between us: the question of which political choices to make. I never managed to think of the irrefutable response here either.

Sam improved people's lives through both medicine and politics, which was his unshakeable and lifelong commitment. And he enriched the lives of those who knew him.

We were lucky to know him and I was lucky to work for him. Remembering Sam always.

Hilda Butler

Secretary, Member of Parliament's and Member of Scottish Parliament's Constituency Office, 1988–2000.

16

The Doctor in Him Made Him the Politician He Became

Alistair Darling

Sam Galbraith was an unlikely politician. I first met him in the summer of 1987. Like me, he was standing for the Labour Party in the general election that year. Unlike me, he managed to avoid the interminable training courses and styling sessions organised for us as candidates. He was too busy in the operating theatre or scaling another mountain.

It's hard to believe now, but thirty years ago the Tories held seats like Strathkelvin and Bearsden, where he stood, with comfortable majorities. And Michael Hirst, the incumbent, was then a respected Member of Parliament. I faced a similar mountain in Edinburgh Central. As did our mutual friend, Brian Wilson, in Cunninghame North.

In truth, none of us really expected to win until halfway through the campaign, when it was clear that middle Scotland was turning away in deep disenchantment from the Conservative Party. It was to be another decade before something similar happened in England. Sam had the biggest challenge. Labour had come third in the seat in 1983. But all three of us won comfortable majorities.

Today, it's often said that MPs lack a hinterland. You could not say that of Sam. By the time he stood for Parliament he had established a world-renowned reputation as a brilliant young neurosurgeon; he had a strong academic background; he had led mountaineering expeditions to the Himalayas and delivered babies amongst the Inuit peoples of North America.

I was not the only one to ask Sam why on earth he was giving up all of this. His answer was simple. He had achieved a lot as a doctor. But many of the problems he dealt with were symptomatic of wider problems in society. He told me that when he travelled from Greenock where he grew up to Glasgow University, he would reflect on his peers who were never going to go through the portals of that ancient seat of learning. Not, he stressed, because they were not capable, but because they would never have the opportunity.

Here was a man who was driven by the injustices he saw while growing up. He rightly saw no reason why the same skills that enabled him to do so much as a doctor could not be applied to solving the entrenched problems all around the West of Scotland.

The House of Commons, when we arrived there, seemed a strange place. It fascinated Sam in the same way, I suppose, as Sam the surgeon would have been fascinated by a rare tumour on the spinal cord. He threw himself into life as a back-bench opposition MP. His irreverence towards authority and his unorthodox bedside manner caught the attention of not only his colleagues, but of commentators. This was no run-of-the-mill Scottish MP. Here was someone very different, very special. About this time a television documentary was broadcast featuring Sam's work in the operating theatre. How many MPs would have killed for such exposure!

To me, Sam was always more of a natural doctor than a politician. His medical qualities are well documented in this book. Sam's instinct was to examine the evidence and then reach a conclusion based on it. This is not always typical of the political approach.

Sam lacked the guile and low cunning that are so often the

dark mark of politics. What he did have were those rare qualities – authority, which he wore lightly and easily, and respect.

Sadly, 1987 brought news that would overshadow his political career. He was diagnosed with fibrosing alveolitis. He was told he would probably have two years to live. As his physical condition deteriorated, it severely affected what he could do in the House of Commons. With only days to live, he had a lung transplant. It was to give him another 25 years of life.

Ironically, he and I would have been attending a seminar entitled 'How to Be in Government', organised by the Labour Party for shadow ministers, on the day of his surgery. The seminar proved to be premature.

Sam had not expected to survive. The birth of his first daughter came just before his surgery. He did not think he would see her grow up. She is now a successful doctor herself. And there were two more girls to see flourish and achieve. They, with Nicola, were the light of Sam's life.

Sam returned to Westminster after several months' recuperation. His spirit, indomitable at the worst of times, was even stronger. After the general election of 1992, it was clear that unless the Labour Party changed and began to appeal to the middle ground of politics, not just in Scotland but throughout Britain, we would never win the power needed to change our country for the better.

Although Sam had been tempted by the short-lived Scottish Labour Party in the late 1970s, he had soon rejoined the Labour Party and was always what is now referred to as a moderniser. This was not a matter of left or right, but simply a pragmatic understanding that a Labour Party which is unelectable is as much use as a surgeon without a scalpel.

He was close to Donald Dewar. He, like me, backed John Smith. On his untimely death, many of us agonised over choosing between Gordon Brown and Tony Blair in the leadership election. I remember Sam was one of the first to say it had to be Tony. He, Sam said, could reach out to the millions of voters we needed to win back; not just in England – middle Scotland exists too. Sam knew that well – Strathkelvin and Bearsden had its fair share of leafy suburbs, just like so many constituencies south of the Border. It had been persuaded to vote Labour and so could they.

In 1997, following Labour's landslide victory, Sam was appointed Health Minister at the Scottish Office. He told me at the time how much he valued the opportunity to make changes. He enjoyed having access to civil servants who were a world away from the 'Yes Minister' stereotype. The respect was mutual. When Sam died, a senior civil servant told me of the palpable shock felt as news of his death spread amongst her colleagues. There was a genuine affection and deep respect for a good man and a fine minister.

In two years at Westminster, Sam was able to demonstrate what a good minister can achieve in office. He had found opposition frustrating – understandably so. Sam brought to bear his experience and authority as a doctor to change policy. The scale of his ambitions at this time are set out elsewhere in this book. However, at the heart of his approach was the recognition that health is to a large extent conditioned by the environment in which we grow up.

Sam was not afraid to confront his former medical colleagues. I know he found it frustrating at times but he was able to face them down, drawing from his armoury of humour and the fact that he knew what he was talking about. Too many ministers from all political parties have found themselves bamboozled by the fact that they are up against the medical profession who have an inbuilt respect from the general public. Sam had no such problem.

He was, though, always reluctant to sell himself or his policies. In an age where presentation often trumps policy, Sam was adamant that the facts and the evidence would speak for themselves.

The conflict between Sam the surgeon and Sam the politician was acutely illustrated in the summer of 2000 when he was responsible for education at Holyrood. The quango charged with marking exam papers – the Scottish Qualifications Authority (SQA) – was embroiled in a row over grades. The day before the news broke, Sam and I, with our children, were on my small boat in the Hebrides. Actually it had been Sam's boat which he'd kept on Loch Fyne, but which he sold to me as his health made it more difficult to handle.

As we floated on a very calm summer's evening, enjoying a beautiful Hebridean sunset, Sam told me that when the SQA published the exam results the next day, all hell would break loose. He said that there was a rational argument to explain what had gone wrong, but that understandably the response of young people and their families to the uncertainties created would be deep anger and frustration.

I said to Sam: 'You're telling me all of this in a boat, and tomorrow morning the solids will hit the fan.' We both knew he had to get on the front foot, and discussed whether he could do that in interviews from Lewis or whether he would have to go back down to Glasgow. It was clear that in his head Sam knew that, but he was desperate not to have to drag Nicola and the girls away from a much-needed and long-awaited few days' holiday. Time was precious to him.

Sure enough, next day all hell broke loose in the media. Sam had the phone wedged to his ear, dealing with the fall-out. He knew television interviews were needed and that reassurance was necessary. Unfortunately, the fact that he did the interviews from a Hebridean island outraged some of the commentators. Why wasn't he in Glasgow or Edinburgh?

Sam said to me: 'For goodness' sake, I'm in Scotland.' If there was ever an example of a good man traduced, this was it. Nor was the affair helped by the fact that Sam had no suit with him. He appeared instead in his holiday ensemble of an old Harris tweed jacket. It was not well received in the West End of Glasgow.

The family departed the next day for Glasgow. I felt for Sam. It's difficult to convey to anyone who has not been through it how vicious and irrational the media and commentators can be. It is of little comfort that the same people can praise you to the skies once they are sure you are not coming back.

Sam recovered from this episode. He was resilient. But his health was not good. We could see the increasing strain was taking its toll physically. For his own and his family's good, he had to get out. He decided to retire from not only Westminster, where he had continued to represent Strathkelvin and Bearsden until the general election, but also from Holyrood, in May 2001.

By this time, Sam had decided for his family's sake that his health would be better served by retiring from the gruelling world of politics. I saw him a lot after that. I sensed he was much happier within himself. I think he found that being a politician – being in the public eye – was more difficult than he had feared. He went back to life as an academic. He could not operate but he could and did advise younger surgeons.

He took up the fiddle with a vengeance. Fortunately the house had thick walls. And he sat on various social security tribunals – something he enjoyed. A year before he died I rang him on a cold winter's night. Nicola answered the phone to say that Sam had been sitting in a tribunal in Hamilton. He had left for home just as snow began to fall. He was now stranded somewhere on a motorway in the West of Scotland.

Here was a man who was reputed to be the world's longest

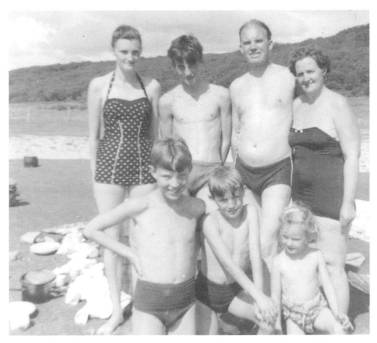

The Galbraith family on holiday at Ostel Bay, Kilbride, Argyll, August 1959.

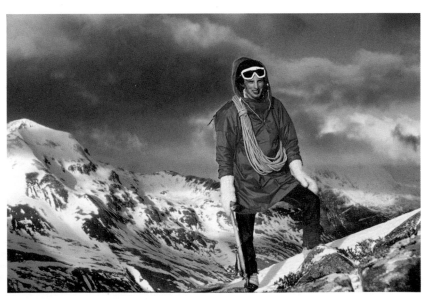

In the mountains: Ben Nevis, 1970.

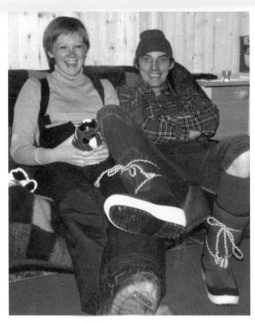

'Happy Days', Sam and Nicola in Val d'Illiez, Valais, Switzerland, 1981.

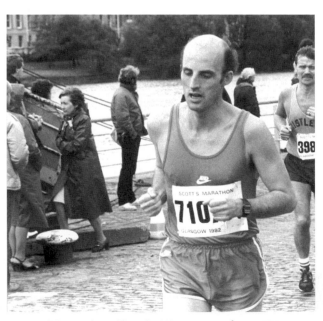

'Hitting the wall' at the Glasgow marathon, 1982.

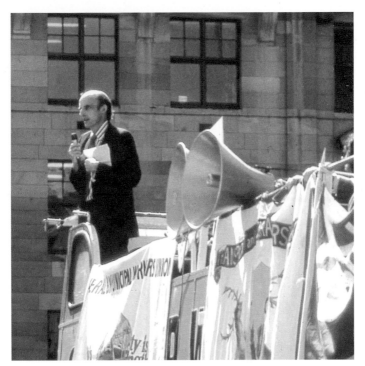

Speaking from the health care workers' campaign bus, George Square, Glasgow, 1982.

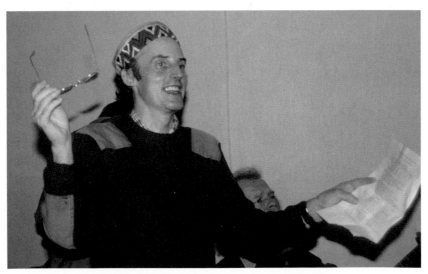

'Oh, my big hobnailers', Leckelm, Ullapool, 1985.

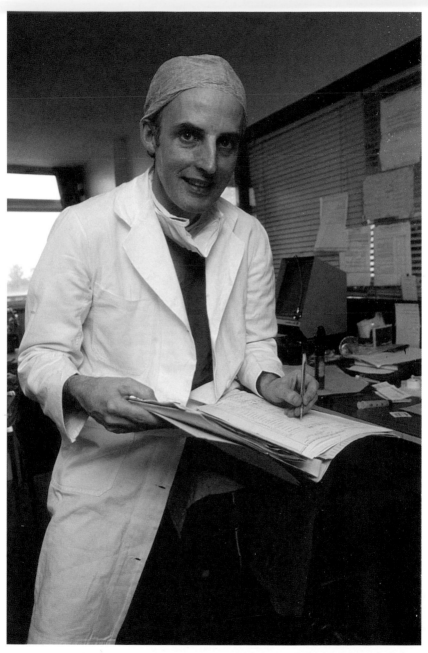

Consultant Neurosurgeon, Institute of Neurological Sciences, Southern General Hospital, Glasgow, 1987.

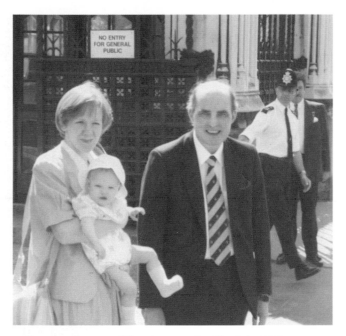

Return to Westminster en famille, *July 1990.*

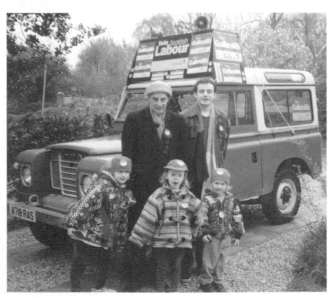

Sam and Jonathan Butler with three junior canvassers and the venerable Butler Land Rover, 1997.

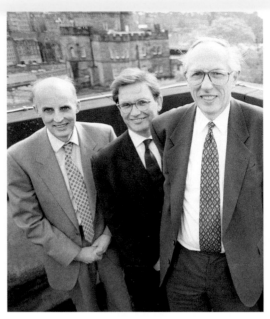

Sam, Brian Wilson and Donald Dewar: New Ministers in the Scottish Office, May 1997.

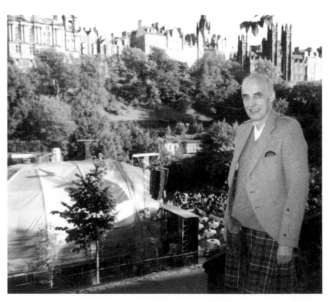

'There shall be a Scottish Parliament', Edinburgh, 1 July 1999.

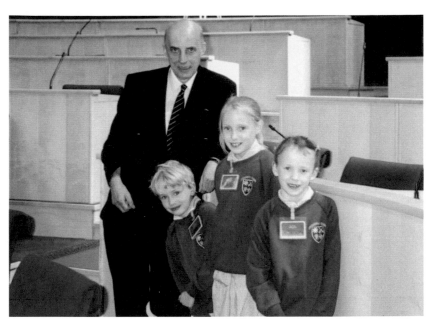

'Checking out the Chamber' of the Scottish Parliament on the Mound, Edinburgh, 30 June 1999.

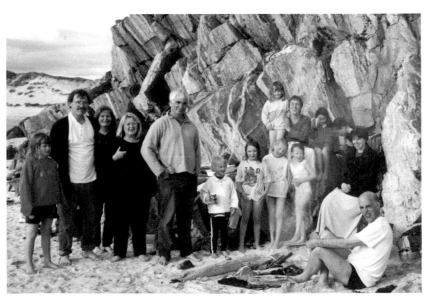

Barbecue on the beach at Little Bernera, Lewis, with the Wilsons, Darlings and friends, 2000.

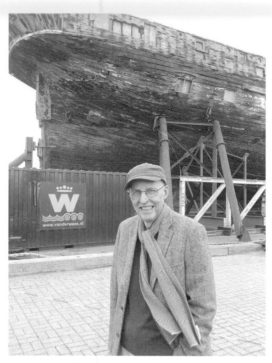

In front of The City of Adelaide, *Irvine, the Scottish Maritime Museum, in 2012.*

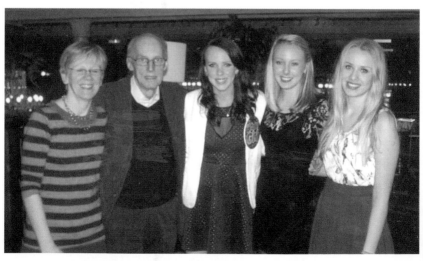

Nicola, Sam, Heather, Mhairi and Fiona, January 2013.

surviving lung transplant recipient, waiting for a snow plough to dig him out. Luckily he had his ancient tweed deerstalker in the car.

Sam maintained his interest in politics, with the occasional trenchant public comment where he vented his frustrations. He was not fit enough to do as much as he wanted in the referendum campaign but he kept in touch with me, offering advice and critique of the nationalist case, some of it repeatable.

In his last interview, he made an eloquent and compelling argument for staying in the UK. When he had his lung transplant, he went to Newcastle, the world-renowned centre for transplant surgery. It didn't matter where you lived, there were no questions, it was there for you. To Sam, whose entire political philosophy was based on sharing, pooling knowledge and expertise, it seemed farcical to break up the NHS because of a geographical border.

It is so sad that he didn't live to see the result of the referendum.

As I look back on Sam's life it's important to understand how much his family meant to him. Our children are of similar ages. We were older fathers. But the days we spent with each other's families in Sam's wee chalet on the shores of Loch Fyne or on the beaches of Bernera in the Western Isles, were amongst the happiest of days.

Sam's grisly humour, and such a happy family, made our visits memorable. He drew tremendous strength from Nicola and the girls and his wider family. Still today, I often think to myself, 'What would Sam think?' His maturity and depth of thought, his humour, particularly a dark humour we shared, were a joy and remain an abiding memory.

I will always treasure thoughts of sitting with him, with a glass of malt, in front of a roaring peat fire in the Hebrides. Sam was a brilliant doctor and neurosurgeon, he was a teacher, and an inspiration to so many people from every walk of life.

The doctor in him made him the politician he became. He achieved so much in his life and could have achieved even greater heights, but for his health. Sam Galbraith has left his mark. He is gone now but I hope others will read his story and follow him. Scotland desperately needs people like Sam to shape our future.

Alistair Darling

Labour Member of Parliament, 1987–2015; Chancellor of the Exchequer, 2007–10.

17

Managua to Mangersta, via Westminster

Brian Wilson

I think I first met Sam in Miami Airport. As he came through the arrivals lobby, he accorded me his traditional greeting: 'You're overweight.' We were both involved in a fine little organisation called Scottish Medical Aid for Nicaragua, a poor country trying its best to establish a democratic government of the left. Sam led fund-raising in Scotland to build and staff a health centre which gave me my initial first-hand measure of the man.

Our visit to Managua was a revelation in many ways. Sam noted with glee how some of our very left-wing colleagues did not take kindly to the basic accommodation at their disposal. He, of course, was better accustomed than they were to the hair-shirt and mountain bothy. As always for Sam, the only consideration was not his personal comfort but the job in hand. He revelled in pricking pomposity, from whatever quarter, and visiting his own uncompromising brand of humour upon those whose words and deeds did not quite match one another.

Before that time, of course, I had known him well by reputation. He was the brain surgeon who marched for the nurses; the consultant who insisted that he was only one of a team, and who was known to all of them simply as 'Sam'; the trade unionist whose day job was to save lives in the most urgent of circumstances; the arch-advocate of Britain's National Health Service. I also knew personally a surprising number of people who owed their lives to Sam's surgical skills – and that alone made him stand out from any crowd.

This was in the early 1980s and by then, Sam had reached the fundamental conclusion that he could achieve more for a greater number through Labour politics than as an individual doctor, however eminently qualified. That was a highly unusual perspective, which was in due course guaranteed to make him that relatively rare specimen – a politician with a specialist interest and agenda, who really knew what he was talking about, from many levels of personal experience.

In that period, there really was an ideological threat to the NHS which had to be countered by people of Sam's calibre and commitment to its essential principles. In Scotland and beyond, he became an inspirational witness in that battle of ideas. Privatising large chunks of the National Health Service was not just wrong in principle, but incredibly inefficient in the use of scarce resources. Sam was able to argue that case not only on the basis of his work within the UK but also from having seen other systems in practice, particularly from his time in Texas.

These were desperate days for Labour, and for some of us the options seemed stark – either become involved in order to help sustain the Party's mainstream, or else see it destroyed as an electable force on which so many people depended. From our different routes, we made the same choice. Sam and I entered the House of Commons together, quite literally, on the same day in 1987. We travelled down together, and just as we were about to pass through the Members' Entrance for the first time, we were tipped a wink by Norman Godman about two adjacent desks whose previous occupants had lost their seats.

They were in what was grandly known as the Cloisters, but anywhere else would have been called a corridor. And there we squatted for a couple of years, until the time when Sam became ill. We also briefly shared a flat in Bethnal Green, but that was an ill-starred venture. It was sparsely furnished and Sam declared that he would go out to buy some essentials. He came back with three radios – and nothing else. We soon went our separate ways to more congenial surroundings.

On his first day in the Commons, Sam was approached by one of the tail-coated attendants in the Members' Lobby whose job was to hail MPs who had messages to collect. He told Sam that a colleague of ours, who was not of the medical fraternity, had advised him that he wished to be addressed as 'Doctor'. Knowing Sam's background, the attendant asked if he would like the same form of address. 'Naw, naw,' said Sam, 'I'm far too senior for that.'

Sam was never overawed by celebrity or reputation. In fact, sometimes he didn't even recognise it. A journalist friend of mine, Duncan Campbell, was – and still is – in a relationship with the actress Julie Christie. One night not long after becoming MPs, a crowd of us went out for a meal and Sam was sitting opposite Julie. After a couple of convivial hours, there was a lull in the conversation and the unmistakable Galbraith tones rang out for all to hear: 'And what do you do yourself, Julia?'

The first signs of Sam's illness had emerged following the 1986 expedition to the Himalayas, where the gallus intention had been to conquer a hitherto anonymous peak and name it 'Partickhill'. But the legacy of that adventure turned out to be grimly serious. His condition deteriorated to the point, in 1989, where he knew that only a transplant would save him and that he was involved in a race against time. It was only with days to live that Sam received a lung transplant at the Freeman Hospital in Newcastle, which continued to provide him with such magnificent treatment for the rest of his life. After the operation, he spent a period of recuperation with Nicola and their infant daughter Mhairi at our home in Lewis, and memories of that tranquil retreat never left him. He loved the West Highlands and Islands, for their beauty, for their peace, above all for their mountains.

Eventually Sam returned to the fray and built a reputation as a diligent and much-respected MP, applying the same humane concern to the needs of his constituents, wherever there was genuine need, as he had become accustomed to with his patients. Ten hard years of Westminster opposition were scarcely suited to Sam's condition but he persisted – away from home during the week, late-night sittings and the inevitable sleeper journey back to Glasgow. If Scotland is a village, then that sleeper buffet car was the main street on Thursday nights and everyone knew Sam. Sometimes, he lived such a full and normal life that it was tempting to forget the seriousness of his condition – a mistake, of course, which he never made himself.

When Labour won in 1997, Sam became Health Minister in the Scottish Office under Donald Dewar. For him, it was the best possible job – the chance to make a lasting difference to how the NHS was run in Scotland and to apply the wealth of knowledge he had acquired through practical experience over many years. It was a time when the NHS had suffered much uncertainty and Sam was the ideal man to affirm basic principles and restore morale. He was a very good and decisive minister and I would bet my bottom dollar that every one of the strategic decisions he took about the use of NHS resources and priorities has stood the test of time.

It was unusual for a minister to have such an elevated professional reputation directly related to his brief. This meant that Sam had a very clear view of how he thought the Health Service should develop and be improved upon. It gave him an authority to resist the kind of populist campaigns to which health ministers are inevitably exposed. It is easy to save a local hospital and leave others to live with the resultant waste of resources for decades thereafter. Sam could respect the good intentions behind such campaigns but was disinclined to succumb to them, in the interests of short-term acclaim, if the case did not stack up. Saying 'no' as a politician is much more difficult than saying 'yes', but Sam was better at it than most.

He won the respect of the people who worked for him in government through that willingness to take hard decisions and by force of argument rather than simply by asserting his status, whether medical or political. Sam's capacity for flippancy and outrageous banter never concealed the fact that he was deadly serious about his political objectives which, above all, were about transforming the life opportunities of those who had been dealt the weakest hands. It was they who needed not only the best possible health care but also the changes to environment and lifestyle which otherwise reinforced their disadvantage. For Sam, the links between poverty, poor educational opportunities and subsequent low life expectancy were self-evident.

Sam was a convinced devolutionist and one of the few MPs who joined Donald in the transition to the Scottish Parliament. Probably more than any other minister in the short history of Holyrood, he understood the potential which devolution created for doing things differently in response to distinctively Scottish circumstances and expectations. That was the whole point of it. While others might worry about getting too far out of line with what Labour was doing elsewhere in the UK, Sam took the view that that was up to them – but this was how it was going to be in Scotland. Even though he did not continue as the Health Minister once Holyrood was established, he exerted considerable influence over the development of policy, particularly through the emphasis on public health.

Sam worked closely and loyally with Donald Dewar through the hasty process of fulfilling Labour's commitment to establish a Scottish Parliament. He was also undoubtedly better aware than the rest of us that Donald's own health was declining quite rapidly, and that he suffered constant pain and discomfort from his back disorder.

The Scottish media's vicious, petty treatment of Holyrood in its formative days distressed Donald and, I think, sickened Sam who could see the corrosive effects of this mindless vendetta at close quarters and from his own very distinctive perspective. People like Donald and himself had battled hard and long, with great personal sacrifice, to establish a Scottish Parliament. Now it was there, they found that they were given no time or leeway to make it work effectively for the Scottish people, before the sharks circled in search of easy pickings. For as long as Sam remained in politics, he continued to make a difference for the better, but he also knew when it was time to get out.

After standing down as an MSP and in spite of his uncertain health, Sam maintained an incredibly full life. But there was one outstanding priority for the years that remained to him, and that was, with Nicola, to raise Mhairi, Heather and Fiona to adulthood; a mission which they fulfilled with such spectacular success. When the end came, our sadness and sense of loss at Sam's passing was tempered by gratitude that we – and much more important, his family – had him for much longer than might have been the case.

Sam and Nicola came to Lewis as often as they could. A plaque on the wall of our very rural local surgery bears his name from ministerial days. Not only was it in Lewis but the GP was a great mate of his from Fort William days – what better reasons for a ministerial visit? Then the last time he visited us in Uig was when he and Nicola arrived for the 21st birthday of our son Eoin, who has Down's Syndrome. They had been with us every step of that journey and Sam, whatever the personal challenge, was not going to miss that occasion.

We remember Sam, not primarily as a politician or a doctor, but as the kindest and most humane of friends who truly made a difference. And who knows how overweight I might have become, if it was not for his regular insults?

Brian Wilson

Labour Member of Parliament, 1987–2005; Founding Editor of *West Highland Free Press*, 1972.

18

He Was Really on the Side of 'the Wifeys'!

Maria Fyfe

'Wifey Fifey'. That was Sam's nickname for me. I think it was for two reasons. One, I was the sole female Scottish Labour MP when we were both elected to Parliament for the first time in 1987. Two, I made a habit of taking up what he called 'wifey' concerns. Well, there were worse nicknames for Hon. Members that succeeded in capturing some element of the victim. Probably everyone now knows who was the Member for Baghdad West.

Both Helen Liddell and I have been called Stalin's auntie – or granny. Indeed, any Labour woman who is remotely assertive is liable to be called that. To which the only answer is: 'And don't forget it!'

Sam's name for Helen was 'Nelly'. And just to see if he could get a reaction, in the taxi queue late at night, more than once he sang a ditty to the sand-dance tune whose words went something like this:

'Does your ma drink gin, does she drink it from a tin?

Nelly put your belly next to mine.'

Not that Helen's composure was to be dented by anything like that.

He laughingly confessed that one day his daughters, pupils at Jordanhill, were singing that song and a teacher reproved them saying: 'That's not a nice song. What would your Daddy say if he heard you singing that?' To which they replied: 'It was Daddy that taught us it.' Sam was very proud of his daughters and their successes, and told his friends how glad he was he had managed to survive to see them grow up.

Any time I did anything that Sam found 'wifey' he was sure to comment on it. When John Smith was off sick with his first heart attack I was convener of the Scottish group of Labour MPs at the time. Naturally I thought it appropriate to buy a get-well card and have it signed by as many members of our group as I could find. Luckily, that very night we were having a meeting. The card I found seemed just the ticket. It had a cartoon depicting numerous wild animals running around dementedly, with the caption: 'We can't menagerie without you.' So, as Sam signed with a cheerful message and passed the card back to me, he commented: 'That was a wifey thing to do.' 'Are you really telling me,' I replied, 'that if I wasn't here not one of our 49 men would have thought of it?' Then he said: 'Probably. Women are much nicer than men.'

'I used to be arrogant,' he told me. 'When I visited my patients at their beds, as I did my rounds I would wave dismissively at all their get-well cards festooned around their beds and say: "Never mind all that. I'm going to get you well."' But now after being seriously ill himself, when it was he who was lying in the hospital bed, he realised how much benefit there was psychologically in receiving lots of cards from anyone and everyone who cared enough about him to do that. 'Honestly, Sam!' I replied, 'The "wifeys" with far less education than yourself, sitting at the hospital bed visiting their sick friend or relative, knew that.' But at least he did now.

There was something else he didn't know that surprised me. For some years Sam, Lewis Moonie and Donald Dewar shared the flat on the landing opposite me in a refurbished block in Kennington. Only Lewis was confident about using the washing machine. I pointed out to this brain surgeon, doctor and law-yer that such machines were designed to be operated by people who couldn't pass an O-grade. They spent fortunes in the local laundrette, and Sam expressed the view that the way to avoid ironing shirts was to buy non-iron ones. Well, that was better than another Glasgow Member who posted large envelopes full of his shirts, pants and socks to his wife. I had always doubted the notion that men couldn't multitask, but when they asked me how I could find time to wash and iron my clothes, and I replied it was easy – you could think up questions or write speeches in your head while handwashing or ironing – they remained dubious. I had had a husband, two sons, and worked most of my life in jobs where men were in the majority, but this degree of ineptitude – in people elected to run the country – floored me. Then I realised it was just a ruse to get out of doing boring little tasks.

On a winter morning, Donald would offer me a lift in his ministerial car that had come to pick him up. One morning, earlier than usual, I heard a loud knocking on my door. I was still in the shower, but as somebody seemed to be in an almighty hurry I wrapped my bath towel around me and went to answer it. Sam was peering through the door window, and called to me, 'You're not going out like that, are you? It's freezing out there.'

But I must record how Sam could be an absolute stalwart when it came to women's health. Toxic Shock Syndrome is a potentially fatal illness that needs urgent hospital treatment when symptoms develop. There had been instances of women dying because they did not recognise the symptoms until too late. Over-long insertion of a tampon is one way the illness can suddenly flare up, and there was a need for education and clear guidance on the tampon packets. When Jo Richardson and I took up the issue of toxic shock syndrome, and I gained the opportunity for a Ten Minute Rule Bill, there were men in the

Commons who felt that subjects such as that should not be discussed, let alone have a Bill being debated in the Chamber requiring appropriate action from the manufacturers of tampons. 'What is this place coming to?' Nicholas Soames cried aloud. Jo and I had meetings with the manufacturers, and to forearm ourselves with medical authority we consulted Sam and other doctors in the House. But it was Sam who agreed to attend these meetings with us, and backed our cause. In the end the manufacturers came round without legislation even being debated any further. Clear warnings would now be put on the packets.

When abortion rights were being debated, to describe Sam as forthright would be an understatement. On one occasion a supporter of SPUC (Society for the Protection of Unborn Children) was describing the details of how surgical abortions were carried out, and saying such procedures were horrible. To which Sam replied: 'Of course it's horrible. It's horrible when you saw off a man's leg and chuck it in the bin.'

Then came the time when John Smith made me Shadow Spokesperson on Health in the Scottish front-bench team. And I knew next to nothing about health issues. I didn't like to bother Sam, who had a great deal else on his plate, but when he saw my first effort at creating a fact booklet for campaigning he looked it over and put me right on a point where I had been mistaken. I had assumed a drop in hospital bed numbers was a bad thing, but he pointed out that advanced surgery had made it possible to let patients go home sooner than before, hence fewer beds were needed in particular wards. And of course everyone knows that nowadays mother and baby leave the maternity ward far sooner than previous generations did. I always thought it a pity that when Sam went to the Scottish Parliament, Donald Dewar made him Education Minister instead of giving him Health. He would have been an enormous asset to us in that role, but

Donald wanted him to broaden his profile by acquiring expertise in other fields.

Sam and I were frequently in disagreement about policy issues, but there was one thing on which we emphatically agreed. In earlier days, back in the '70s, we had joined Jim Sillars' Scottish Labour Party. Both now regarded that as an embarrassment we hoped others did not know about or had forgotten. When it came to the Scottish referendum we could have competed to be the most committed No voters in the land.

Sam was generally known as one who didn't mince his words. He would be likely to dismiss an argument with 'Away and bile yer heid.' An official of the GMB, the boilermakers' union, at the conclusion of a lobby of MPs, remarked of him: 'He talks mair like a bilermaker than a bilermaker.' Which was true. Refined was not the word for Sam.

Then there was the Children (Scotland) Bill. It had been twenty-five years since there had last been any legislation about children in Scotland, and the Commons had only recently updated child law for England and Wales alone. As one of George Robertson's deputies on the Scottish front bench, I was put in charge of our side for the committee stage. I found some of my male colleagues were dubious about their ability to contribute, and I had to persuade some that they were needed to make up the team. But Sam stepped up to the plate immediately. His presence made a great difference. When Tory ministers at first refused a request from me, Sam confronted them and suddenly there wasn't any problem. A little male aggression came in handy.

That committee did something that has always been within the rules, but seldom applied. We called in a variety of organisations that were relevant to children's lives to advise us before debate began on the clauses in the Bill. They could comment on the draft Bill, and make fresh suggestions of their own. In turn the committee members, regardless of political party, found this particularly valuable, learning more than they had ever before about the dreadful lives some children led, and changed the law to benefit children accordingly.

Sam was an assiduous attender at these meetings, questioning and probing. Then when we went into committee it was a delight to hear Sam comment on 'wasters' – men who ran away from their responsibilities as fathers, and didn't pay their fair share of their children's upkeep.

When Sam went off to the Scottish Parliament that did not mean losing touch. A few of us old mates from our House of Commons days formed the 'Last of the Summer Wine' lunch club, and meet occasionally for a bite to eat and talk of, what else but politics. Despite failing health he took on new responsibilities after he retired from the Scottish Parliament, and got along to join us whenever he could. Of course he never failed to put a view intended to outrage me, just for fun. But that was Sam. We miss him.

Maria Fyfe
Member of Parliament, 1987–2001.

19

The Confidence to Do Things Differently

Kevin Woods

I first came across Sam Galbraith when I read an article in the *British Medical Journal* about his maiden speech to the House of Commons in 1987. In those days I was making my way in NHS management in an English health authority, having been a student of health politics in an earlier academic career. The article caught my eye because of what Sam had said about the need for better management systems ('business principles applied primarily to delivering patient care, not saving money'). These ideas resonated with me, but little did I realise that ten years on I would be working with Sam after his appointment as Health Minister for Scotland. I have always felt that the convergence of our paths in St Andrew's House was a matter of great good fortune for me as it opened up one of the most enjoyable and creative phases of my own career.

On the Tuesday after the 1997 general election, Sam met with the then NHS Management Board. Like a lot of ministers taking up post he wasn't sure what to expect of his civil servants, and he could be forgiven for being suspicious about a group of people who had served Conservative administrations over many years and which had very different ideas about the NHS. At this first meeting something unexpected happened. When Sam, with his newly appointed private secretary, entered one of the art deco meeting rooms on the third floor of the Scottish

Office, the whole group of senior officials stood spontaneously. In retrospect it probably reflected recognition of Sam's achievements in medicine, and respect for the courage he had shown in continuing his political career after his lung transplant. A few days later Sam greeted a senior official with a beaming smile and proudly announced he had the key to the ministerial lavvy! There were no airs and graces with Sam. We all knew that we were about to embark on a period of wholesale change. Proposals rapidly emerged which have a continuing impact to this day. They included plans to change the operation of the NHS; plans to achieve equity in how resources were distributed to different parts of the country; plans to reorganise acute hospital services and introduce new arrangements to quality assure clinical care; and plans to improve Scotland's adverse health status.

Tony Blair's New Labour election manifesto had set out plans to 'modernise' the NHS. A core commitment was to end the internal market, introduced by Margaret Thatcher's government and her Scottish ministers in 1989, with the creation of NHS Trusts and GP fundholding. As an aside, I recall Sam saying that he thought the adoption of the name NHS Trust was a clever idea, but he also thought that the internal market had to go and go quickly. He did not like GP fundholding. He saw it as a distraction with the risk that it could distort the delivery of the best patient care through bureaucratic contracts with hospitals driven by short-term financial incentives. But he could also see that it had led to the engagement of energetic and enthusiastic family doctors in innovative practice which he did like, though on the whole he had an unjustifiably low opinion of general practice. Early on I said to him that we knew what he wanted to abolish, and that we knew he did not want to return the NHS to the world pre-Thatcher, but we were not sure what he wanted instead. His answer was: 'That's for you to work out.' This was a remarkable invitation.

In 1997 most policy in Scotland reflected Westminster policy. The NHS was no exception, but with the prospect of political devolution and the creation of a new Scottish Parliament in the offing, things began to change. In the six months between his appointment and the publication of *Designed to Care*, the White Paper which set out his plans for the NHS in Scotland, Sam demonstrated an independence of spirit and a determination to do what he thought was right for Scotland's health service. He obviously enjoyed the confidence of Donald Dewar, and no doubt there were many private discussions about the way ahead, but I can only remember the Secretary of State attending one briefing on the White Paper when we were asked to explain its proposals. He signed up to them. That they differed substantially from the plans in England was of no evident concern to Sam, not least because in the period of their making it became very obvious that English ministers were not intending to abolish the internal market after all, merely repackaging it. Similarly, Sam did not have the same enthusiasm for presentational matters as did some in Whitehall, believing that if the substance of policy was right the presentational issues could be sorted relatively easily. An energetic Wendy Alexander played a prominent role as the White Paper neared completion, but Sam was very clear that political special advisers were not to get in the way of officials working to him on the policies.

Alongside proposals for health services, a wide-ranging consultation on how to improve population health was undertaken, leading in 1999 to the publication of the White Paper *Towards a Healthier Scotland*. It proposed action focused on life circumstances, lifestyles and health topics, with an emphasis on tackling health inequalities. As a result of his clinical career in Glasgow, Sam had first-hand knowledge of the adverse effects of social deprivation on the health of Scotland's poorer communities and was determined to do something about it. The significance of this work should not be underestimated, for previous administrations had never given them any priority, at one time being suspected of trying to bury the publication of a landmark study (the *Black Report*) which made uncomfortable reading for them, highlighting – as it did – the scale and consequences of poverty on health. Health policy in Scotland has subsequently had a continuing focus on these matters, so the ideas in *Towards a Healthier Scotland* mark a turning point as important as *Designed to Care* was for health services.

Around the same time, a review of the public health function in Scotland was undertaken under the direction of Sir David Carter, the Chief Medical Officer (CMO), for whom Sam had great respect, both as a clinician and public servant. Its central ideas were that health boards should be 'public health organisations' and that 'health in all policies' should inform wider government policy-making. Ultimately this led to the creation of a Public Health Institute for Scotland (PHIS) only for this attempt to strengthen public health leadership to disappear subsequently into the inner workings of Health Scotland, a special health board.

For a man with his personal medical history, Sam showed remarkable energy, though he once asked a nurse showing him round an Ayrshire Hospital to 'slow down love, I've only got one lung!' Only once, while a minister, do I recall him being concerned about his health. On a visit to Aberdeen Royal Infirmary he sought some assistance with his medications, but it didn't hinder him in any way. He travelled the length and breadth of Scotland and its health services, and everywhere he went he seemed to know someone from his earlier medical career. He didn't stand on ceremony and was renowned for his propensity to dispense personal health advice to those he met. Despite its potential to cause offence he seemed to get away with it, and not only because he was the Minister; it was Sam's way, and most took it in good part. Greeting a colleague from the past he said something like, 'You've put on a bit of beef,' and on another occasion told a local NHS leader that his weight was incompatible with his role running health services, although put more bluntly along the lines of 'You really are a fat cat.' It was said without malice and with a twinkle in his eye.

On a more serious note, Sam had a complex relationship with the profession to which he belonged. He found himself in a lengthy row with the leadership of the BMA in Scotland. It was sometimes felt that he was judging them as doctors first and as professional representatives second. If they did not measure up against his professional yardstick he could be critical of the message and the messenger. Most of the rows were about the pressure on hospital services, especially but not limited to the Edinburgh Royal Infirmary. Reports of patients waiting far too long in the A&E department received prominent coverage, and neither side of the argument minced their words. For the BMA its Scottish Secretary claimed that the hospital was in crisis; for its part the hospital acknowledged there had been lengthy waits, but its medical director denied that there was a larger crisis. The BMA's Secretary had described the Royal Infirmary A&E as a 'war zone'. The Minister replied, 'I am fed up with this scaremongering . . . there has been a silent revolution in the Health Service. Some people have not left their rhetoric behind but we have moved on. The NHS in Scotland is not in crisis. I am disappointed that comments by one union official on a visit to one hospital is regarded as a comprehensive survey of the state of our NHS.' (*Glasgow Herald*, 7 January 1999). The use of the word 'union' rather than, perhaps, 'professional body' was deliberate. It was Sam's way of displaying the contempt he felt for some of the BMA leadership over this issue.

There was another strand to the conflict with the BMA, and that was over the funding of new hospital developments. There was an urgent need to rebuild many of Scotland's major hospitals, and, in common with other parts of the UK, Labour ministers embraced the Private Finance Initiative (PFI) model initially developed by the previous Conservative governments. It was controversial. Some believed it would open the floodgates to the privatisation of the NHS, others that it was a financial three-card trick which would ultimately leave the NHS with unmanageable burdens of debt, and others were worried that the hospitals would not have the required capacity for the forecast demand. The BMA had a lot to say on all of these points, and it was undoubtedly a tricky issue for the Scottish Office.

Ministers' attitude to PFI was soon tested. If there had been any doubts, they were soon dissipated by the approval of four major hospital building projects (Hairmyres and Law Hospital in Lanarkshire; a community hospital in Ayrshire; and the largest of all, the Royal Infirmary of Edinburgh in August and September 1997) (*Hansard*, 3 July 1998, col 277). Sam did not like PFI, but planning for these schemes had been under way for many years and it would have been impractical to abandon them or find the amounts of money required from public sector capital budgets. Sam even went to Stonehaven to officially open the Kincardine Community Hospital, a controversial project conceived and agreed before his time, which at one point might have led to the privatisation of some clinical services. This was a red-line issue for Sam. If confirmation was needed, however, these early decisions demonstrated that PFI (relabelled as Public Private Partnerships, PPP) were now firmly part of NHS policy in Scotland, a demonstration of New Labour's pragmatism, summed up as 'What matters is what works.'

One of the responses to the pressures facing hospital services between 1995 and 1997 was an urgent examination of acute hospital planning assumptions. Undertaken for the Conservative government of the day, it recommended a wider review of how Scotland's acute hospitals should be organised, and the incoming government supported it. Led by the CMO, Sir David Carter, this review generated some far-reaching proposals, expansion of cardiac surgery and a new focus on health care in Scotland's remote and rural areas amongst them. But the most significant were ideas to establish hospital networks, to assure clinical quality, and to separate elective and emergency hospital treatment in the form of Ambulatory Care 'walk in, walk out' services. This last idea was the subject of special funding to the tune of £2 million to allow experimentation, but subsequently turned into the building of the new Stobhill and Victoria Hospitals in Glasgow (at a cost of many millions more!).

Managed Clinical Networks (MCNs), sought to reconcile the benefits of local access with the benefits derived from the concentration of clinical expertise. MCNs were defined as 'linked groups of health professionals from primary, secondary and tertiary care, working in a coordinated manner, unconstrained by existing professional and health board boundaries, to ensure equitable provision of high quality clinically effective services throughout Scotland'. The concept was rapidly adopted in Scotland and elsewhere.

The Acute Services Review's proposals for the quality assurance of clinical services were implemented by the creation of the Clinical Standards Board for Scotland and its successors (NHS Quality Improvement Scotland, and now Healthcare Improvement Scotland). If this was the obvious organisational consequence of the Review, the accompanying development of 'clinical governance' within health services was of as much or perhaps even more significance. It is hard now to think of an NHS without clinical governance processes, but that was the case at the end of the 1990s. Sam appropriated a definition of clinical governance as 'corporate accountability for clinical performance', the significance being that it brought the quality of clinical practice, hitherto the preserve of the medical profession, to the centre of the governance responsibilities of health care organisations.

Against this background Sam got to grips with the problems of Glasgow's acute hospitals. There was an urgent need for new investment in them, but agreement on what should happen at each of the six major hospital sites was elusive, creating a political minefield which frustrated progress. Sam cut through this, undoubtedly exploiting his first-hand knowledge of Glasgow hospitals and his clinical standing. He understood the implications of developments in science, technology and clinical practice and their complex interdependencies. According to those closely involved at the time, Sam never proposed his own pet solutions or interfered with the flow of conversations in Glasgow, but he always showed a keen interest in progress and would offer his own pithy observations about the credentials of the naysayers who bedevilled the process as it unfolded. The process lasted many years and involved many committed people in Glasgow and beyond, and all of Sam's successors as health ministers. But today Glasgow has an outstanding system of high quality acute hospitals which stands comparison with any in the UK.

It is very rare for ministers to combine such expertise, enthusiasm, encouragement and support on a personalised basis. His own clinical background undoubtedly gave him confidence to interpret the direction being taken. Since his comments were based on personal clinical experience they had a magnified effect in giving confidence to the NHS people locally who were putting their heads above the parapet in promoting change. In the words of one person closely involved at this time, 'Sam didn't just give a green light, he constituted the pole star, shining brightly above us all, which gave us confidence in our navigation.'

But there were some ideas in the air that Sam would not embrace. In Clydebank a private hospital (Healthcare International, HCI) had been constructed with substantial public money as part of an industrial development plan. The idea was that the hospital (which had extremely good facilities) would attract patients from the Middle East and elsewhere by capitalising on the clinical expertise of Glasgow's NHS. The venture never really worked, and its owners signalled that they might do a deal with local health boards and bring the hospital into the debate about Glasgow's acute hospitals. The idea was broached in a conversation with Sam Galbraith. He wouldn't engage at all with it. He took the view that HCI should never have existed in the first place and would have no truck with anything that might 'save it' or involve the NHS getting somehow tainted by an association with it. Subsequent ministers took a different view and the hospital passed to the NHS and became the Golden Jubilee Hospital, initially as a national centre for elective surgery, and subsequently the West of Scotland centre for cardiothoracic surgery.

There were other important policy initiatives in the early months of Sam's tenure as minister. In December 1997 a national review of how to allocate NHS funds to different parts of Scotland was announced. The question of how to divide up Scotland's health funding between its area health boards had become a significant issue, as it was felt the formula for dividing the cake was outdated. On the one hand rural and remote health boards complained it failed to take account of their increased costs, while others complained that it failed to take proper account of the effects of social deprivation on the need for health-care funding. Professor Sir John Arbuthnott, Vice-Chancellor of Strathclyde University at the time, was invited to tackle these problems, a task to which he devoted a great deal of time and energy in his long and distinguished career. The product of this work was the publication *Fair Shares for All*. Sir John has described how he came to be appointed after Sam approached him at a charity dinner in Glasgow, and subsequently in London, when Sir John recalls Sam with his feet on his desk reflecting on the job to be done. The implementation of the review fell to those who followed Sam, but it might not have happened at all without Sam's willingness to confront the problem.

The NHS enjoyed its 50th anniversary in 1998, and various events were held to celebrate it. The centrepiece was a service held in St Giles Cathedral in Edinburgh, and he and Donald Dewar took a close interest in all the arrangements. But the event that mattered most to Sam was the idea of the Scottish Fiddle Orchestra giving a performance at the Glasgow Royal Concert Hall. Those involved in the practicalities were introduced by Sam to the leader of the orchestra who had links with the Institute of Neurosciences in Glasgow, and they recall Sam and his family sitting in the front row entering fully into the spirit of the occasion.

When arrangements were made for Wiseman's Dairies to put the NHS 50th anniversary logo on its milk bottles, it caused high anxiety at the most senior level of the Scottish Office administration lest it be seen as an official endorsement of a particular milk supplier. Sam agreed with the actions of the officials involved and resisted the concerns. Such actions made Sam popular with those who supported him during his time as Minister, and many officials recall their engagement with him with obvious pleasure. There have been many talented ministers before and after, but Sam's personality, his prestige as a distinguished surgeon and a very special patient, won him many admirers in the Civil Service. Some especially enjoyed the freedom he gave them to create policy. If there was sometimes the feeling that he could have given more direction, that was an acknowledgement of the value his experience and insight could offer. For all who worked with him, Sam's time as Minister is remembered, as is he, with affection and admiration.

Kevin Woods

Director of Strategy and Performance Management, 1995–2000, later Chief Executive of NHS Scotland, 2005–10; Director General of Health, New Zealand, 2011–13.

I am grateful to former colleagues who have shared their memories of Sam as Minister and helped to inform this chapter.

20

The Civil Service and a Relationship Built on Mutual Respect

John Elvidge

Would Sam have described us as friends? Probably not. We shared some interests and some values, and there might be some similarities in parts of our personalities, but ours was essentially a working partnership.

Sam did not have any of the personal insecurity visible in some ministers, which would have led him to look for displays of personal admiration from civil servants. Quite the reverse – he was well able to describe his own strengths as a minister.

He was right about what they were. He understood that the most effective ministers know their own minds and are enthusiastic about taking decisions based on their judgement of the arguments. He would point out drily that neurosurgery is not a profession for the indecisive.

Our paths hadn't had much reason to cross in Labour's first year in government after the May 1997 general election and, by the time I returned at the point of devolution in May 1999 from a year or so in the Cabinet Secretariat in Whitehall, Sam had built up two years' experience as a minister. So it was he who had to live with me settling into my new role as Head of the Scottish Executive Education Department, rather than the more common reverse process. I had every reason to be grateful that he was fully confident in his role and that he was content to give me time to adapt my experience of overseeing policy and performance across the UK to the more direct responsibility for helping him guide policy and deliver performance in Scotland.

We were both, of course, adapting to the uncharted territory of devolved government. It was not in his nature to ask for help with that and, in any case, I'm not sure that he saw much need to adapt his style. I could not help but reflect, though, on Sam's likely response when I came across newly elected Members of the Scottish Parliament who thought that it was a larger version of a local authority, that Sam was merely the equivalent of the Convener of the Education Committee and that civil servants were as accountable to them on a day-to-day basis as they were to him. Ignorance for which he could see no excuse tended to bring out the more brusque side of his nature.

I think Sam and I were able to get off to a good start because I had established a good working relationship with Donald Dewar, as Secretary of State for Scotland, in the year before my spell in the Cabinet Secretariat. Sam was fiercely loyal to Donald, and my guess is that he took the view that if Donald had a good opinion of my capabilities, that was sufficient recommendation.

Not that Sam was given to suspicion or disrespect towards those who were working to support him as a minister. In contrast to many ministers I have worked with in my various senior management roles, Sam did not bring me a litany of complaints about the work of individual officials. This may have been partly because his approach to being a minister brought out the best in people. His clarity of political direction helped them focus their efforts well and his understanding that you get the best from people by encouraging them made my colleagues enthusiastic to give him the best support they could.

Even the best minister does not magically inspire perfection in every civil servant. As an example of a minister who has had a life before politics which involves having oversight of the performance of others, Sam understood that some variations in ability are a fact of life in large organisations and he knew that the best way to deal with lapses in performance was to be straightforward and to make clear the standards he was expecting.

If he did not agree with advice or was unpersuaded by the way policy was being put into practice he would say so plainly and explain his misgivings. His intellectual rigour was never far from the surface of his dealings with people and he was at home alongside a civil service culture which takes pride in the coexistence of robust argument and good personal relationships. He knew that he would never be short of allies in reinforcing the standards which mattered most to him.

His tolerance of human fallibility and freedom from pomposity extended to circumstances which would have tried the patience of many people. We had adjoining offices with less than perfect sound insulation. One afternoon I was dealing with some tensions between the relatively junior staff who supported me and those tensions erupted into raised voices. After a while Sam appeared at the door and asked if there could be less noise. The chastening effect lasted a little while but the volume gradually rose again. Sam did not reappear to reinforce his message more robustly nor did he do what many ministers would have done and send someone from his own office to deliver that message. Few ministers would have been so understanding, but perhaps this was another example of the fact that he was familiar with the occasional trials of overseeing the working relationships of teams of people.

I worked with Sam in both of the two cabinet minister roles which the Department supported. He was the first Minister for Education in the devolution era and the second Minister for Culture and Sport.

The event which divided his two ministerial roles and which caused the transition to happen was the most intense challenge of our time working together: the SQA crisis in the summer of

2000. Sam was caught in the eye of that political storm, despite the fact that it was not of his making and there was nothing which he could reasonably have done to prevent it. His vulnerability to the media and political pressure for him to be the scapegoat, rather than the Board or Chief Executive of the SQA, illustrated two aspects of his political style.

His belief that rational argument and a proportionate view of the facts should prevail was ill-matched to the understandably emotional nature of the responses by young people and their families to the uncertainties which the SQA was incapable of resolving. He had no great repertoire of media-handling tricks, not least because he had no desire to be that sort of politician.

He was also not one to turn to special advisers for such tricks. He held very strong views about the place which they should occupy relative to ministers, and the respect he showed for others was sometimes replaced by dismissiveness when he was dealing with those whom he regarded as having a distorted view of the fundamental difference in authority between the two groups. There was no trace of the courtier in Sam's nature, and it was not a set of behaviours which he had regard for in others.

This approach to those whose position within government rested solely on ministerial patronage was consistent with his strongly traditional view of accountability. For him, a proper view of ministerial authority went hand in hand with a willingness to take responsibility for the things which happened within his span of authority. That view of ministerial accountability made him willing to take responsibility even for things which he could not have controlled. He was unusually free from a preoccupation with allocating blame.

I was a beneficiary of that. When the first indications of problems emerged and I and my colleagues were just beginning to establish the facts, Sam was on holiday with his family in the Western Isles. We were in daily phone contact and I said to him that there was no aspect of the problem at that stage which could not be dealt with adequately over the phone, and that I had no reason to ask him to leave his family and come to Edinburgh. He was rapidly criticised for not rushing back from his holiday, but at no point did he blame me, privately or publicly, for not giving him better presentational advice.

His attitude to remitting office as Minister for Education, as it became clear that media and political pressure around the SQA's failures of competence was not abating, reflected his clear view of ministerial accountability. Whatever he felt about it, there was no trace of self-pity or complaint in the way he communicated it. He simply turned calmly and professionally to his new role as Minister for Culture and Sport. He also recognised without rancour that my priority at that time had to be supporting Jack McConnell, as his successor, to bring the SQA issues to a successful conclusion. For him, it was an issue about wanting the team to do well, and wishing Jack less than complete success would have been alien to his strong sense of loyalty. I think Sam would have disdained the word 'comrade' because of those who used it insincerely, but he certainly knew how to behave like one.

My memories of our time working together in his new role are also mainly dominated by his knowledge of and empathy for the cultural side of his responsibilities. Alongside that there are also sharp memories of our biggest crisis. Scottish Opera had got itself into serious financial difficulties and had precipitated the series of events which eventually required the company to go dark for a period as part of the rebuilding of its financial stability.

Despite the existence of the Scottish Arts Council to make decisions about the funding of individual companies, the problem was rapidly in Sam's lap and therefore also in mine. Sam simultaneously demonstrated both his deep knowledge of and affection for this major element of Scotland's cultural scene, and a clear determination not to excuse failures. In a period when the focus of others often appeared to be interpreting the past in such a way as to absolve themselves of blame, his priority was to get to a solution in which everyone shouldered their future responsibilities. He channelled any frustration he felt with individuals into a slightly more terse version of his usual decisiveness when dealing with them, but, as ever, he made the strength of his views clear without the tantrums in which some of his ministerial colleagues indulged themselves.

I remember the same control of emotion in Sam from several other key moments, for example when he explained to me the cause of Donald Dewar's tragic early death, at a time when it was still very raw for everyone and particularly deeply felt by Sam. Or when he called me into his office to tell me that he had decided to step down altogether from ministerial office. On the latter occasion, it is one of my lasting regrets that his own calmness led me to miss the best moment to tell him how much I had enjoyed working with him.

Like a number of others, I have his present of a Willie Rodger print to remember him by, and have been cheered to have it prominently displayed in my various offices through the rest of my working life. I also draw upon his outstanding example of public service to keep my optimism buoyed up when I hear the virtues of public service denigrated or denied.

Sir John Elvidge KCB

Head of Scottish Executive Education Department, 1999–2002; Permanent Secretary to the Scottish Government, 2003–10.

21

The Holyrood Years

Jackie Baillie

Where to start? So many thoughts and memories flood my mind that it is difficult to know where to begin when thinking about Sam Galbraith. From my time as the Constituency Party Secretary when we selected Sam Galbraith to be the Scottish Labour candidate for Strathkelvin and Bearsden in the 1987 general election, I have been very proud to call him a friend. Confining myself to his years in Holyrood will therefore be hard.

A sharp intellect; a dry wit; an enormous sense of fun; cheeky and direct, are just some of the comments people would make about him, which gives you a sense of how he did his business. Heaven help you if you were on the receiving end of his merciless teasing. Driven by deeply held values of social justice and fairness, he was passionate about his politics, a committed advocate for his constituents and, above all else, devoted to his family.

As one of the class of 1999, Sam was an important member of the Scottish Parliament. He brought with him experience of UK politics and government, having been appointed as Minister for Health and the Arts in the Scottish Office by Tony Blair when Labour came to power in 1997. He did not however wield his Westminster experience too overbearingly, recognising that this was a new Parliament with an opportunity to do things differently.

Perhaps of greater significance was his friendship with Donald Dewar. He was in my view the best friend that Donald had in the Scottish Parliament. Fiercely loyal to him, Sam expected others around Donald to be loyal too, and he could be quite scathing of those guilty of doing the opposite. He hated the culture of briefing against each other that existed in the Party at that time, particularly amongst members of the Cabinet.

No one more than Sam tried to help Donald adjust to the demands of national leadership as well as leading the Scottish Labour Party in the Parliament. It was a tough time at the start, as all of Donald's energy had been focused on legislating to create the Scottish Parliament while running the Scottish Office and winning the first-ever elections to Holyrood. The criticisms from the press at the time suggested we were unprepared – having created the institution, we did not appear to know what we wanted to do with it. Sam was constant in his support and advice to Donald and helped to refocus our efforts.

He was a source of support, encouragement and advice to many of us as brand new politicians, most holding ministerial office for the first time. I well remember his words to me – always do what you believe to be right and that will see you through the toughest of times. And it is as true today as it was then.

Although he would never let on that he was disappointed, many of us strongly believed that Sam should have been given the health portfolio in the first Scottish government. A brilliant neurosurgeon, Sam knew the Health Service in Scotland inside out. We all say that Scotland is a small place and, in that context, the NHS is a village. NHS staff all knew Sam well, and he had a huge regard for them too. He understood the challenges facing the NHS and he was seized of the opportunities to make it better for patients and for staff alike. This was evidently all too challenging for the Civil Service, to have a minister who knew his brief much better than they did, and I believe that they had a hand in convincing Donald Dewar to appoint Sam to education, rather than health.

Sam would never admit that he wanted the health role and I have to say that he made a really good fist of the education brief. With young children himself, Sam would bring his lived experience about what mattered to parents directly to the heart of the portfolio.

In his time there Sam brought forward the Standards in Scotland's Schools etc. Act 2000. He worked within quite difficult financial constraints to oversee the biggest expansion of classroom assistants ever, alongside training up a new generation of teachers. I remember, as a mother of a seven-year-old at the time, having engaging conversations with Sam about expanding nursery provision and affordable flexible childcare, as he juggled with his own family commitments. It brought out an altogether different side of Sam and he would be quite animated about the possibilities. Surrounded by an all-female household and with every one of his private secretaries being a woman, I used to joke with him that we would make him an honorary sister. It was the ultimate compliment that I could pay to him, and an accolade I think he secretly quite enjoyed!

Sam had his share of challenges to deal with in the portfolio. I recall in particular the problems with the Scottish Qualifications Authority (SQA) and exam results in 2000, when thousands of students received inaccurate or incomplete results. Sam and his officials, time and time again, sought assurances from the SQA which were given and subsequently proved to be worthless. In handling the problem, he was clear who was to blame and what was needed to put it right, and he did not shirk from doing so. His manner and professionalism reassured us all. At the very forefront of his mind were the needs of the young people, their families and teachers who had worked so hard and deserved to have their efforts properly recognised.

And who can forget: 'Trust me, I'm a dad. I wouldn't do anything to harm our kids.' That was when Sam was tasked with bringing forward guidance for schools when my ministerial colleague, Wendy Alexander MSP, announced that Section 28 was to be repealed. Section 28 had been put in place by the Tories to prohibit any discussion of homosexuality in schools and removing it was a simple matter of equality for almost all parties across the Parliament. Sam's task was undoubtedly the most delicate faced by any politician in the first Scottish government. In the face of a vitriolic counter-campaign, Sam's calm assurances struck a chord with parents, and he managed to balance the interests of all who put forward legitimate concerns, by bringing forward guidance that is still used today. He was quite simply superb at getting people to move forward and agree.

And he had Hampden Park and Scottish Opera to deal with as well. All was done with his usual direct, no-nonsense approach. In November 2000, Sam moved to a new portfolio of Environment, Sport and Culture, all the things he loved combined together. He took Donald Dewar's death very badly and civil servants close to him remarked that they had never seen Sam so frail. He had lost much more than a political colleague, he had lost a friend. Frank as ever, he made it clear he was not continuing under Henry McLeish unless he got a portfolio with things he enjoyed.

Those last few months as a cabinet minister saw Sam visit museums, galleries, sports grounds and some of Scotland's most beautiful locations: lochs, mountains and national parks. He was one of Scotland's hardest-working ministers and this was undoubtedly a labour of love.

When he announced he would be stepping down, many of us were very sad. Watching his BBC interview with Gordon Brewer on his last day as a government minister, some of us shed a few tears. This was truly the passing of an era. I often wonder, had Donald lived and Sam stayed on, would the Parliament have been a better place? There is no hesitation in my mind: the answer is yes.

I want to end this chapter by making you smile. Sam was a warm and caring human being but he was incredibly cheeky and far too direct for his own good. He got away with murder. There is a saying 'to know yourself as others know you' . . . So here is a collection of stories from politicians, private secretaries and press officers that offer us a little insight to Sam. Some were just too rude to print, but all at their heart contain a real fondness and admiration for the man that was Sam Galbraith.

Sam had nicknames for everyone – his private secretaries, Sarah Davidson, Rachel Sunderland, Gabby Pieraccini and Katy McNeil were all endowed with 'Big' or 'Wee' in front of their names according to their height. His press officer, Murray Meikle, was called 'Luggsy', and every time Sam had a spare few minutes he offered to use his surgical skills to 'pin his lugs back' for him. Mike Ewart, Director of Education at the time, had a crew-cut. Sam would summon him by shouting, 'Get me Bullet-Heid!' And he never referred to George Foulkes as anything other than 'Fatty', while I was always asked, 'How's the diet coming along?' Just as well that I liked him!

I was also reminded by the government car service drivers of his comments to Helen Liddell when they shared a government car from Dover House to catch the flight back home on a Thursday evening: 'Come on, Nellie, get yer erse in the car!'

It is to his private secretaries that I turn now, for they deserve the final word. As one told me, Sam started every morning in the office with a roll and fried egg. This was usually to be followed by locating a spare tie. He would try to embarrass his private secretaries at every opportunity, when not trying to give them the slip. I am sure that GPS trackers were often talked about.

They tell me that he liked nothing better than walking down

the ministerial corridors in George IV Bridge or at Victoria Quay with civil servants trailing in his wake, shouting 'Walk this way!' while putting on a silly walk copied straight from John Cleese.

Seating was something that Sam paid particular attention to – he had his civil servants pinch a big blue sofa from the atrium at Victoria Quay to swap with his own chair because it was too hard. And there was nothing he liked more than the heated seats in the ministerial cars. Indeed he regularly regaled people with stories about the joys of a warm bum.

Always to be found with a bunnet, coat and scarf, he usually handed them to his private secretary and, when departing from engagements after the polite goodbyes, could be heard shouting, 'Where's ma bunnet?'

Sometimes Sam would use the gym in Victoria Quay to stay healthy. He took particular pleasure in terrifying other users who hadn't noticed him. He also liked to plonk himself down next to unsuspecting folk in the canteen and slurp his soup.

When Sam decided he was done at the end of the day, he was off, moving surprisingly quickly for someone with only one lung. 'I'm aff,' he said. 'Wait for your box!' his private secretaries would call. The words 'Bugger off' drifted through the atrium.

There was one occasion when one of his private secretaries needed to call Sam at home. One of his daughters answered the phone and could be heard clearly shouting up the stairs to him, 'Dad, it's the headmistress!'

Sam is remembered as being an incredibly kind and caring man. One of his private secretaries had this to say: 'I spent the first few weeks in private office thinking that he didn't know how to behave as a minister before realising that he knew exactly what he wanted to do and how to be effective doing it. He was a real star and it was a privilege to work for him.'

And this from another: 'The world is a duller place today without the wonderful, kind, sweary, life-affirming former Scottish Minister, Sam Galbraith.'

And so say all of us.

Jackie Baillie

Member of Scottish Parliament, 1999 continuing; Shadow Cabinet Secretary for Public Service Delivery and Wealth Creation, August 2015 continuing.

22

Wise, Rude, Irreverent – and Deadly Serious

Catherine MacLeod

After crossing Westminster Bridge in London with Sam on a dreich March day in 2001, I feared I would never see him again. We didn't walk across, we shuffled, as Sam struggled to make it from one side of the bridge to the other.

At that time I was political editor of the *Herald* and Sam had arranged to meet me because he wanted to announce his imminent resignation from the Scottish Executive, and his Strathkelvin and Bearsden constituency. It was a typical gesture. He loved Glasgow, he was loyal to the *Herald*, and he was going to give the story to me because I was fortunate enough to be his friend.

Over lunch he said he was sad to stand down but he wasn't maudlin and was perfectly matter-of-fact. He had self-diagnosed. He had little choice. His life depended on getting fit and he could not undertake the requisite swimming and walking while carrying out his ministerial duties. Sam had sorted out his priorities. There were four: Nicola, his wife, and Mhairi, Heather and Fiona, his three treasured daughters. He intended to be there for them as long as he could.

Sam was a bright spot in the political firmament. He was wise, he was rude, he was irreverent, he was funny, and deadly serious about everything he considered important. Recognising injustice, unfairness, the iniquities of the system underpinned his politics and the way he led his life.

When I first met Sam in the early '80s he was en route to Nicaragua with his great friend Brian Wilson, who later became an MP and a minister with him in the Scottish Office. They were internationalist in outlook, driven to make the world a better place, whether on their own doorsteps or thousands of miles from home. As head of the charity Scottish Medical Aid for Nicaragua, Sam had raised £60,000 for a health centre in that war-torn country. He believed passionately that health and life-expectancy needed to improve if countries and individuals were ever going to prosper.

In the House of Commons and beyond, speaking to journalists, friends or colleagues, he would recall his feelings as he made the daily trip from his parents' home in Greenock to Glasgow University while his former school mates were not so fortunate. Many had left school at 15 with no qualifications and, therefore, little choice but find employment where they could. Sam often railed against the unfairness of selective education, citing its lasting damage and corrosive effect on individuals and communities. Forty years later he could still recall the names of people scarred by the ignominy of failing the 11-plus exam.

He also never forgot the dire poverty and ill health which existed within the community in which he was brought up, and it is to his lasting credit that he eventually persuaded the powers-that-be of the direct link between poverty and bad health.

These personal experiences underpinned his political life, and what he had to say in private matched his public pronouncements. Sam admired ability, but woe betide the pretentious. Invariably, in Sam's company, whether they were Cabinet members or jumped-up colleagues, they would be heading for a fall. Lampooning pomposity he regarded as sport.

Sam believed the people who needed the most help needed the best political representation. He didn't approve of time-served political hacks ending up in the House of Commons as a career move, and was not shy or afraid to bemoan the intellectual deficiencies of some of his colleagues.

Equally he had little truck with those who held to the belief that surgery was a higher calling than politics. While he had great admiration for good surgeons and health practitioners, he strongly believed politicians and the political process could be a more transformative force for the greater good.

Along with Labour colleagues he trawled the world looking at ways to improve and secure the National Health Service, to discover how other systems worked and what could and should be cherry-picked. His international fame opened many doors, and from what he learned on these fact-finding trips, and his own experience of working in a health service in which money changed hands, his hostility to private medicine was reinforced.

In 1988, not long after the then Labour leader, Neil Kinnock, appointed him Scottish Health Spokesman, Sam confirmed Labour's commitment to absorb private hospitals into the NHS. In government in 1997 he persuaded colleagues to fund areas where the NHS had been letting people down, and drove a campaign to improve Scotland's diet and public health and cut down obesity. There were very few of us Sam did not think overweight.

Sam worked closely with Donald Dewar, one of the few genuine devolutionists in the government. Donald trusted Sam's judgement, respected his opinions and was pleased Sam decided to stand for the Scottish Parliament, to help drive through policies designed to tackle Scotland's health inequalities – though it was odd that Donald did not make him the Health Minister. Sam was not beyond the odd wry observation about devolution. At the referendum count which approved the establishment of the Scottish Parliament with tax-raising powers, he rightly predicted there would be great enthusiasm for tax-raising powers in the areas where little or no tax was paid and less enthusiasm in others.

The National Health Service was a metaphor for how he thought Scotland should be governed: bring decision-making nearer to the people and tailored to Scotland's needs, while also making sure they had seamless access, without any financial consequences or bureaucratic burdens, to resources in specialist treatments, research and training throughout the rest of the UK.

He never resiled from that position, and was a beneficiary of these shared resources when he was called to the Freeman Hospital in Newcastle for a lung transplant. Not only did they save his life but his time in hospital caused him to reflect on the *modus operandi* of consultants. 'I used to think I understood,' he said, 'but you have to be a patient to understand what we put patients through.' He was convinced patients were subjected to too many tests.

Sam told it as it was, and though he expected others to do the same he paid attention only to those he thought had something interesting to say. Only months after Sam was appointed Scotland's Health Minister in 1997, the NHS Management Executive in Scotland decreed there should be no gagging clauses in the contracts of NHS employees, that freedom of speech should be maintained and supported. NHS employees, many of whom Sam had worked with over the years, would have expected nothing less. He understood their value, their contribution to the Health Service and he was their consistent and vociferous champion in the House of Commons and later in the Scottish Parliament. He believed their informed voices should be heard and not shut down by the system and bureaucrats who did not know better.

Politics mattered, and so too did learning, and the hills and mountains which he knew so well.

Nobody understood better than himself the scale of his achievement in the hallowed world of neurosurgery. He was delighted to be a world-class neurosurgeon enjoying the affirmation of his peers, but he didn't conform to any preconceived stereotype of a world-class consultant. With tremendous glee he recounted his meeting with a tourist officer on the Arran ferry. He was returning home after three days' climbing and sleeping in the clothes in which he was standing. He conscientiously answered all the questions, how many days he had been there, what he had been doing, where had he slept and more in that vein. Then she asked him his occupation, and on being told he was a brain surgeon, found the possibility so implausible she scrunched up his questionnaire and threw it away. He loved that.

Often when hanging round the Commons, Sam would be in his element recounting tales of his exploits on the hills, and the times he spent as a young surgeon in the Dr MacKinnon Memorial Hospital in Broadford on the Island of Skye or the Belford Hospital in Fort William. He'd climbed the hardest routes on Ben Nevis, and though he'd led an expedition to the Himalayas and had climbed regularly in the Alps he loved talking about hills in the Highlands, their challenges and the inspirational beauty of the landscape.

If I was standing in the journalists' Lobby, next to his friend Ewen MacAskill, then the political editor of the *Scotsman* and now the defence editor of the *Guardian*, talk of climbing experiences took on another dimension, and politics became very much of a second, third or fifth order. Ewen stands in awe of Sam's courage and determination, and recalls a rock climb he made with Sam many years after his lung transplant. Sam had been despondent, reflecting that his rock-climbing days were over. Ewen thought differently, and off they went to climb the Whangie, a 40-foot rock outcrop in the Kilpatrick Hills near Glasgow, and one that Sam would have completed in his heyday without a second thought. This time he grunted and puffed and vomited on any ledge he found to rest on the way to the top. Ewen says Sam was not being macho: rather it was a demonstration of physical courage and grim determination. Half an hour later they were enjoying a pint in the Carbeth Inn.

Political campaigning with Sam was a surreal experience. Who could forget him in an old folks' home in Ross-shire persuading the elderly residents to limbo dance under a broom handle, he holding one end and the cleaner the other. This was as he implored them to get off their backsides and keep fit. On another visit to an old people's home, Sam was accompanying Donnie Munro on the campaign trail in the Highlands, where Donnie, formerly the lead singer of the Scottish rock band, Runrig, was the Labour candidate. Sam dispensed with the political messaging and demanded Donnie sing *An Ataireachd Ard* to an elderly lady from Lewis. To Donnie's consternation and Sam's delight the image captured by the photographer was Donnie complete with Labour rosette sitting beside an old lady with her eyes closed as if she was bored to tears, rather than transported to the island of her birth by Donnie's beautiful voice.

Sam had the intellectual self-confidence and the medical know-how to plough his own furrow when political policy and health issues collided. His years in the theatre of the Southern General Hospital generated a lifelong horror of boxing and motorcycles. Had his view prevailed he would have banned them both. Boxing he deemed to be no more than assault unacceptable in civilised society, and motorcycling not much better. His description of head injuries after a motorcycle accident would make the strongest stomachs turn.

Regularly he frustrated colleagues and communities campaigning to keep open their local hospitals. While he understood they played an important role in communities, he did not think they were appropriate places for specialist operations. Though it meant the centralisation of facilities, he argued consistently that it was always better to be operated on by an expert rather than a generalist. 'No more bellies being opened in these places' was his mantra. He would ask pointedly who would trust the lives of their children to a surgeon who opened a belly once a month rather than every day of their lives. Few had a suitable riposte.

Whatever Sam's private anguish, he neither sought nor expected warm words. Sitting beside him on a plane back from a weekend in Morocco he instructed me on what I should do in the event of his demise. Nicola was sitting on his other side but he surmised she might need a hand.

My last image of Sam is of him dancing with Nicola at Eoin Wilson's 21st birthday party in the community hall in Uig on the island of Lewis. They had driven from Glasgow, taken the ferry from Ullapool to Stornoway and then dressed up in their finery to suit the Hollywood party theme. They made a particularly glamorous couple.

Catherine MacLeod

Political Editor, the *Herald*, 2001–07; Senior Special Adviser to the Chancellor of the Exchequer, 2007–10.

23

The Galbraith of Galbraith

Angus Macpherson

Oh, we're all so stuffy in the law, and writing about Sam at the General Medical Council (GMC) means betraying all those vows I have taken to preserve confidentiality; and Sam the least stuffy panel member ever, a man gifted with humour, infectious joy, humanity (particularly towards the young) and profound commonsense. It cannot be done.

But I give you a portrait, as best I can, of a man whom I am grateful to have known for a few years. He would greet me with his characteristic opening gambit: 'Is that yourself, Macpherson of Macpherson?' audible to a significant part of the GMC common room and one made in the full knowledge that I was not that esteemed person. At once it was warm and mischievous, and conveyed delight in our encounter. It gave me confidence that we might sustain a friendship and so it proved.

We sat together on perhaps three or four cases, each lasting a few weeks. He was a panellist, one of three; never the chair. I was legal assessor to each of those panels. I can't tell you about those cases, save that they were a mixed bag of clinical issues allegedly amounting to misconduct, and one or two allegations of dishonesty. But I can disclose that his presence punctured self-importance and enhanced the quality of the hearings. He did not, to my knowledge, take much of a note, but was always abreast of the issues which the cases presented and asked salient questions. And then there were the lee periods when the panel awaited witnesses, submissions from counsel or draft determinations and

Sam would talk. Not loudly or boastfully, and not necessarily about himself. He talked with glee about people and matters important to him, about his climbing, about George Galloway and about the things which interested others. He cared about people, especially the people of Glasgow. I understand that it was his concern for their health which took him into politics. In his last case at the GMC, he was still wondering why the people of Liverpool, who had a similar racial mix to those of Glasgow, were blessed with better health.

I learned about his early climbing days and the division of his working week to accommodate this. Monday to Thursday evenings were set aside for work, weekends for climbing. Friday evenings were for other activities. His climbing was not limited to mountains. It extended to scaling buildings inhabited by his fellow students and colleagues, swinging in through windows, depositing or removing things and leaving detected or undetected. Quite clearly he was impish, dangerous and wonderful at the same time. No one could forget him.

I also learnt that he was the Chair of the Scottish Maritime Museum Trust and proud to be so, but he was embarrassed that he had never visited the National Maritime Museum in Greenwich. It so happened that I was organising a clan outing to view the Macpherson Collection of maritime paintings in the Queen's House at Greenwich on 13 July 2013. Sam said he would like to come. It was the hottest day of the year and clansmen were to meet at Westminster Pier at 10 in the morning and boat it down the river. Sam only had one lung. In Manchester where the GMC sits, he used to trudge from his hotel to the hearing venue, wearing a woolly hat and looking for all the world extremely down on his luck; likewise if he was out in the evening. May Nicola forgive me. Here he was proposing to fly down from Glasgow in the morning, get to the pier at the appointed hour, do the trip, visit the museum and return to Glasgow that night.

Frankly I was rather uncertain that he would make the attempt, or indeed should make the attempt, and in truth I had forgotten about him, whilst endeavouring to marshal my clammy clansmen onto the ferry. Then I felt a little tug on my sleeve. It was Sam, looking tiny, in a baseball cap, quietly indicating he had arrived and wanting no fuss. Did my clansmen know that we had been joined by such an illustrious soul? Well I wasn't going to tell them until after a convivial lunch in the brasserie, when a few short sentences were to be uttered. But then I lost him. He was not to be found in the Queen's House, nor in the gardens. He was not in the brasserie. No message on my mobile. Not answering his. No signal. Nothing to be done. The next tug on my sleeve was back at the GMC a week or so later. He'd had a lovely time, loved every minute of it, went round the Cutty Sark and back home. He'd visited Greenwich.

So not much about Sam in the GMC is in that tale. But perhaps it shows that energy and conservation of energy were matters of considerable importance to him. He knew what he would like to do, and set about achieving it. I think that must have governed his attitude to the GMC. He had a contribution to make, he had great experience of the world of medicine and was no respecter of the great names. He would have a view in a case and would express it.

I think he was profoundly grateful that he had the chance to continue to contribute. He had survived far longer than the doctors had given him, survived to see his girls grow up, survived to be with Nicola. Others had not. I recall one morning in the common room he was rather quiet after receiving a message on his mobile. His usual garrulousness, after recovery from the walk from the hotel, was missing. He explained that one of his regular climbing friends – I recall that they were a band of just three – had died, and had been found in his flat after some time. That affected him. Still he was equal to the pleasantries of the panel members as they arrived in the common room, greeting them by name. But it affected him.

He was proud of being a Galbraith and once upon a time had thought of embracing Galbraith clan life. Perhaps he fancied himself as a Highlander and that's why he wanted me to be a chief. In fact he knew something of my clan as he had a house in Newtonmore in Inverness-shire, centre of the Macpherson clan. Newtonmore boasts a wonderful Highland Games which he and Nicola regularly attended. I met them one time up there, after the clan march to the Eilan where the games take place. It's a great event, a Scottish Highland event. And Sam would not be missing it. He was a Greenockian and Glaswegian, a brilliant neurosurgeon, a man who cared for and understood people and who had integrity. He would have been welcome anywhere.

Angus Macpherson

Barrister, Temple Garden Chambers, London, 1998 continuing; Legal Assessor, General Medical Council, 2010 continuing.

24

A Passion for Our Maritime Past

Muriel Gray and David Mann

Muriel Gray: Sam as Chair

It's hard to remember exactly where and when I met Sam, because it seems he had the knack of entering people's lives by osmosis.

Everyone was aware of Sam as the people's hero, surgeon turned politician, and in a village like Glasgow he was always at two degrees of separation, a friend of friends. So meeting him in person for the first time is now a long-lost unrecoverable memory.

But I was particularly fortunate to have spent what I now regard as extra special time in his company after he persuaded me (well, that's not quite accurate), *compelled* me to join him on the Board of Trustees at the Scottish Maritime Museum where he had taken over as Chair. If Sam told you you really should do something, you did it.

Sam knew I had maritime links, having had a father who was a chief engineer in the Merchant Navy and who dragged his children below the deck of every ship to admire the engine room, and so we talked long and often about obscure ships and nostalgic trips down the Clyde. Even knowing how much maritime history meant to Sam, I still wasn't prepared for the unbridled affection and passion he had for the Museum, and more importantly for the people who were running it and had cared for it over the years. 'This is all great,' he said on our first visit, pointing to the exhibits, and then, pointing at some young people hard at work sanding an engine, he said, 'but it's meaningless without them.'

Showing me round for the first time as a trustee, he was like an excited child, thrilled by every object and display, knowing the history and provenance of each and every one, and full of optimism about what we could do and the direction the Museum should take, particularly in its shift into becoming a wider education resource. All the volunteers appeared to know him by name, and in turn he knew exactly what projects they were working on. This is not the norm for someone in high governance of a national institution. It was more like the energy and commitment of the enthusiast.

And yet solid governance was of course one of Sam's many skills, and in the time he chaired the Board the Museum went from strength of strength, winning a grant to repair the roof that effectively saved the Museum. His inspiration and encouragement persuaded all around him to up their game and manage the vision and ambitions he had helped ignite in everyone.

For someone who was supposed to have been 'retired' he did a pretty good impression of a person who was anything but, being fully involved and engaged in a project that so clearly meant an enormous amount to him.

We often drove together to Irvine, with Sam barking directions if there was the slightest deviation from his preferred route, and we had a chance to talk about many things, including his upbringing, his love and pride for his family and his continuing passion about trying to make the world a better place. I consider these conversations a great privilege and still treasure them.

People say Sam didn't suffer fools gladly, but I would contest that. He certainly didn't suffer foolishness silently, but beneath the acerbic dry humour, he was kind, gentle, and never patronising or cruel to anyone, especially not to those demonstrably less intellectually gifted than him, which accounts for 99 per cent of the population. He disliked unkindness and bad manners, and sharp as his tongue could be it was never turned on anyone in anger, only in jest. His chairing was of course impeccable, and he was inclusive, encouraging and effective as he was at everything else.

It was perhaps that combination of human decency and nimble, uncompromising wit that made him such an inspiring leader as well as a delightfully unique person.

He lives on in everything he touched and everyone he knew, and it's hard to walk around the Museum now without hearing him at your shoulder telling you what needed 'a bloody good dust' and barely containing his glee, shouting: 'Just *wait* till you see what we're going to with this!'

We can't replace him, but nobody who knew him will ever forget him.

David Mann: Sam's Contribution to the Trust

Sam Galbraith's first encounter with the Scottish Maritime Museum was a meeting with a delegation led by the Chair, Lord Maclay. The Museum had recently lost key funding and was struggling to stay open, so a case for financial support was put before Sam in his role as Minister for Health and the Arts at the Scottish Office. Although no long-term support was agreed at that meeting, funds to keep the Museum afloat to the end of the financial year, 31 March 1999, were approved, allowing time for a study into its future. Its conclusions were discussed at a meeting between Sam and the Museum's Chair and the then Director, Jim Tildesley, at the Scottish Executive in early November 1999. As a result core funding was secured not only for the Scottish Maritime Museum, but also for the Scottish Fisheries Museum and the Scottish Mining Museum. This was a fantastic show of support by the Scottish Executive for Scotland's industrial heritage. Demonstrating his further support, Sam's first visit to the Museum's Clydebuilt site occurred on 22 November 1999 in his capacity as Education Minister. In later years, Sam recalled how much he had enjoyed his first visit, though dealing with the press and media on the day had been less of a pleasure.

In late 2005, Lord Maclay intimated that he wished to resign as Chair of the Museum. An inspired approach was made to a now-retired politician who had been supportive in the past and had a keen interest in maritime heritage. To the surprise and delight of many, including Lord Maclay and the Museum's Board, Sam accepted and was officially appointed Chair of the Scottish Maritime Museum Trust from the start of 2006, bringing vision, leadership skills and a deep appreciation and love of all aspects of Scotland's important maritime heritage to the post. He attached particular importance to ensuring that the Museum's finances were put on a sound footing and that good governance was established. In return he was supported by an enthusiastic Board and a team of dedicated, hardworking and knowledgeable staff. The staff, in particular, welcomed Sam's impromptu visits and the support he offered, as well as the supply of yum-yums from Greggs that often arrived with him.

Under Sam's leadership, the Museum, with the financial support of the Scottish government, reroofed the historic Linthouse building at Irvine and reopened it to the public with an improved award-winning display, and also refurbished the Denny Ship Model Experiment tank at Dumbarton, creating a striking exterior which houses new displays and interactives. The third major achievement was the successful transfer of the clipper ship *City of Adelaide* to Australia. Sam was exceptionally proud of having overseen the completion of these three major projects. With the improved financial outlook for the Museum, Sam indicated to the Board his wish to stand down at what would have been his last AGM on 3 October 2014. As a result of Sam's support, enthusiasm and dedication the Museum is in a position to go forward with confidence.

Muriel Gray

Trustee, Scottish Maritime Museum Trust; Chair of Governors, the Glasgow School of Art, 2013–16.

David Mann

Director, Scottish Maritime Museum, 2013 continuing.

With acknowledgement for input from Dr Harold Mills CB, Vice-Chair, Scottish Maritime Museum Trust, and Jim Tildesley, retired Director of the Museum.

25

Benefits System Tribunal Member

David Hamilton

I gave Sam a reference to assist his application, in retirement, to be a SMQTM (Senior Medically Qualified Tribunal Member) in the Tribunal Service, Scotland, dealing with the appeals from those turned down for state benefits. I was already a panel member and was careful with my reference. The reason was that, earlier, Sam had supported me for my appointment and with his tongue in his cheek wrote that I was 'a determined, lifelong friend of the underprivileged' which was exactly what the Tribunals did not want. What they want are persons of experience and balanced judgement, and Sam brought these to the Tribunals, with his insider knowledge of the political system and experience from his constituency work.

The hearings deal with disability, incapacity for work and industrial injuries. A doctor, a lawyer, and for some types of appeal, a member with expertise in disability, hear from those initially turned down for benefits. This Tribunal work may appear from the outside to be worthy, but routine; instead it is much more interesting. For Sam it proved to be not just an agreeable post-retirement role; there was added political interest. Sam joined at a time when concern about the benefits system was rising rapidly and it was heading upwards on the political agenda, with the Conservative government pointing to the puzzlingly marked increase in disability and taking the view that the availability and levels of benefits discouraged many from seeking work. The definition of disability, and hence for making awards, was also changing. This was based on a tick-box menu, some of the boxes were being removed, and there was a major controversy over the new medical examination system, crucial to the award decision, run by a private firm. Sam was now at the sharp end, watching the operation of the benefits system closely, and he did not support it uncritically. A side-issue was that we knew that the lawyers we worked with had a deteriorating financial position, notably after the cuts in Legal Aid, and that their annuity/private pension prospects were shrinking. Sam, if not indulging in *schadenfreude*, could certainly reflect on the irony of this. When he was involved earlier in the battles about private medical practice, some doctors called for 'professional freedom' and to be paid like lawyers. Sam retorted that the doctors should instead be content with their secure NHS posts and salaries, to which is added a generous state-provided pension.

The Tribunal sessions were formal, but Sam resisted putting on a good suit to impress those attending with the majesty of the law and the mystique of the medical profession. His brightly coloured socks, however, won approval from the women. He did reluctantly remove his signature woolly hat, which was not a fashion quirk, but essential protection for his almost bald scalp which was regularly developing the light-induced skin cancers which are a complication of long-term anti-rejection treatment.

The other Tribunal members soon got used to his style, which was open, relaxed and disarming. Because of this, he was a favourite with the lawyers and he was good at explaining medical diagnoses and jargon in lay terms to the others on the panel. Tolerant of all members of the human race, Sam had a knack, repeatedly commented on by others, of putting the appellants at their ease at this stressful interview, and drawing out from them what they came in wanting to say. He used humour and, with his knowledge of the various trades, not only from his constituency work but also from his early days in Greenock, he could establish rapport in this way. His questioning was focused, speedy and to the point, using earthy everyday words for intimate bodily functions. As ever, his robust language risked offending those of a delicate or touchy nature, but he got away with it, the response being 'Sam is Sam.' Far from offending the appellants, the opposite seemed to be the case. If a Tribunal appeal is turned down, a further appeal against this refusal is generously always possible, and it was noted among the lawyers that hearings involving Sam attracted fewer of these appeals, as if the appellants felt that justice had been done, and had been seen to have been done.

In the discussion after hearing the case, and before the decision, he was decisive and the lawyers noted his impatience with legal niceties, such as the law's affection for debating the nuances of the meaning of words, for instance the difference between 'regular seizures' and 'frequent seizures'. In moving towards a decision, he could also be as sceptical of the evidence as anyone else. He would say so. Just after he started, tape-recording of the proceedings (but not the discussion) was brought in, and the lawyer-chairman often forgot in the early days to switch off the microphone before the discussion began. Sam's blunt assessment, then caught on tape, might cause a sharp intake of breath. On these occasions, he was doubly justified in his scepticism since, in spite of having only one lung (someone else's and by now somewhat damaged), and being personally significantly disabled, he continued to lead a full life.

One little contribution which I tried to spread about in our little Tribunal world was 'Sam's 33/250 Law' which related to his disability. You get state benefit if you claim you can't walk 50 yards before stopping. The medical textbooks, surprisingly inattentive to disability, offer no help on these matters, for instance in estimating the walking distance likely with different grades of a lung affliction. We needed help. Sam's lung function was only about 33 per cent – one third of normal – and Sam could walk about 250 metres before resting (as a government service we had to use the metric system). Our claimants with chest problems, notably chronic bronchitis (COPD), might have function only slightly reduced to 80 per cent yet claimed to be unable to walk 50 yards. Sam was not impressed, and his 'Law' helped.

We had training sessions for the Scottish panel members from time to time and Sam could contribute in his usual incisive way, notably with nippy remarks during dull presentations. One speaker, dealing with the law on mental health, and needlessly brought up from London, announced that 'I believe you have a different system up here.' Sam didn't like the patronising 'up here' and interjected: 'Yes, I drafted the legislation.'

Sam was active in this appeals work right to the end. He sat on a session in Hamilton two weeks before his death, having first presented his colleagues there with self-picked chanterelle mushrooms. He was a favourite with all the staff, and he left his mark.

David Hamilton

Lecturer, later Consultant, Department of Surgery, Western Infirmary, Glasgow, 1971–2004.

26

The Great Venture: Lung Transplantation

Paul Corris

Referral, 10 August 1989

'Go on, go on, leave me breathless.' – The Corrs

'Mr. Sam Galbraith is a local Labour Member of Parliament and prior to the last General Election was a Consultant Neurosurgeon at the Institute of Neurological Sciences in Glasgow. In February, 1987 he presented with an infection and radiological changes of pulmonary fibrosis. He is now significantly breathless.' Thus began the letter of referral to the Newcastle Lung Transplant Unit from his physician Neil Thomson in August 1989.

In 1986 the Cardiac Transplant Surgeon, Chris MacGregor, a Scot who had also trained in Glasgow, as it happened, had knocked on my door as a newly appointed senior lecturer and consultant respiratory physician and asked me whether I was willing to help him establish a lung transplant service in Newcastle. It was a no-brainer, and after reading the very small amount of published literature on the topic and a visit to Toronto to see how it was done, we set about writing protocols and planning the programme. It was still a time when, with the permission of the hospital's chief executive and a chat with relevant people at the Department of Health, innovation in health care could be undertaken by committed and driven people relatively free from stifling governance requirements. There remained an air of 'courage to fail' in the pursuit of novel approaches, providing the plan passed the common-sense test and looked to offer advances in health care with acceptable risks to patients.

We duly performed the first successful single-lung transplant in 1987, and over the next two years steadily built up a reputation as a competent clinical service. This reputation led to increasing referrals from all over the UK, explaining why the letter from Neil Thomson arrived on my desk. By this time, Chris had left Newcastle for the Mayo Clinic in the USA and had been replaced by John Dark, a cardiothoracic surgeon working in Edinburgh who had received training in transplantation at Harefield and Toronto, with previous cardiothoracic training in Glasgow.

Sam was duly seen as an outpatient initially, so we could advise him of our current, and indeed the world's, experience of short-term outcomes and expectations for single-lung transplantation in patients with progressive idiopathic lung fibrosis – a condition of unknown cause characterised by lung scarring. I say idiopathic, but in fact in Sam's case it was familial disease, with his sister having undergone heart-lung transplantation at Papworth Hospital, Cambridge, as a result of the same condition. His sister had developed complications relating to the immunosuppression, so Sam and Nicola were aware of the potential pitfalls and risks of lung transplantation. By this stage it was clear he had rapidly progressive disease that was unresponsive to the immunosuppressive therapy available at that time, and death from respiratory failure within the next year or so was inevitable. He was between a rock and a hard place. Accepting the opportunity for salvation or otherwise by the knife was his choice.

He was straightforward and easy to speak to. He wanted clear matter-of-fact information and expected to be treated as any other patient. It was made clear that was our expectation also. We hit it off from day one, though I wondered right from that moment how easy it would be for him to be in the patient role.

Sam was admitted for full work-up, i.e. a series of detailed investigations and discussions to establish his suitability to undergo lung transplantation, on 23 October. He arrived firm in the view that his disease had progressed to the stage where he should be placed on the active waiting list. He handled the factual medical information well, but he had less time for the discussions regarding the handling of stress and other imponderables. He knew he would cope with stress as he always had. He was a neurosurgeon after all.

I believed I knew him better after that week. I liked him. I enjoyed his dry and not so dry humour, even when I was on the butt-end of it!

Tests of the function of his liver showed that although it was able to carry out the vast majority of its important functions, he had a tendency to jaundice. Specialist hepatic advice was sought and given. 'He freely admits to overindulging in alcohol, but no more than the average medical. I feel confident that Sam does not have liver disease, rather a biochemical abnormality.' He had Gilbert's disease, a benign inherited condition, if truth be known.

There was a short meeting of the relevant transplant team to finalise decisions on candidature (his suitability for surgery) and operation. The multidisciplinary team (MDT) was small in those days and everybody present had met Sam. Perhaps that is a lesson for today's MDTs, which to my mind sometimes lead to decisions by an entire committee best made by a smaller group. There was a unanimous decision to accept and list. I went to convey the decision to Sam and Nicola and advised that in our view Sam should be listed immediately. They both agreed and thanked the team. Later I pondered. I hoped. I wrote to his physicians. Get the paperwork done whilst fresh in the mind. He was listed for left or right single lung transplantation. Sam had balls, Nicola had courage. I liked them.

Surgery, 5 January 1990

'If I chose how to die I would die by the knife.' – Steve Harley

Left single-lung transplant was carried out by Colin Hilton assisted by John Dark on Friday, 5 January. The surgery was precise and uneventful and Sam's new lung began to work well immediately. There was a single pulmonary vein but no other surprises. He was transferred to the Intensive Care Unit and ventilated overnight.

On 6 January I arrived early for the morning ward round.

Sam was awake and had a pleading look in his eyes. I recognised the message: 'Get this bloody tube out!' Blood gases were fine. Chest X-ray was fine with no signs of early rejection or damage relating to infection or adverse effects of the operation. Pain control was good.

My decision was to extubate immediately and it was done. First hurdle cleared. I spoke with Nicola and conveyed the promising news. Nicola and Sam had a young daughter, Mhairi, born in the preceding August. A complete family to bring up children remains best in my view. No added pressure on us then!

Shortly after extubation Sam asked to speak to me. 'I was awake during the operation,' he said, 'I remember the words spoken by the anaesthetist.' I was somewhat staggered.

I spoke with the anaesthetist. 'Impossible,' he said. He spoke with Sam. He was even more staggered. Sam clearly had heard the subject of his conversation whilst under anaesthetic. We should have written the case up as the first lung transplant performed under conscious sedation!

I always advised transplant recipients, and still do, that having a lung transplant is like being hit by a truck on the motorway, being scraped up off the tarmac and transferred to ITU and then resuscitated. I had made no exception when speaking to Sam. 'Yes, yes,' he had said. Now he began to realise how hard it was. He had always coped before in his life as a person by taking control. Now he was a patient. He adapted. He progressed. He had two early setbacks relating to episodes of acute rejection, but these responded well to pulsed corticosteroids given repeatedly intravenously in very high doses.

He had a further setback. Sadly his sister died of complications following her heart-lung transplant. The mood was sombre.

By 8 February he was ready for discharge home to Glasgow. Second hurdle cleared. There was laughter and unabated joy all around the Unit. I reflected on many of the conversations I had with Sam and Nicola over the preceding weeks. He was really a pussy cat with elephant skin. I liked them both. I hoped above hope he would do well. Luck did, and still does, play a role in success, but the harder you work at it the luckier you get.

Readmission, 15 February 1990

'If you don't eat you don't shit, and if you don't shit you die.'
– Australian saying adapted by Paul Corris

Sam was admitted having presented to Glasgow with severe malaise, fevers and breathlessness.

He felt dreadful. He looked dreadful. He progressively became worse. The diagnosis was reactivation of infection with a virus called cytomegalovirus, CMV for short. This is similar to viruses responsible for chicken pox and glandular fever, but can damage the digestive system, lungs and eyes after transplantation.

We gave him passive therapy with an antibody, CMV hyperimmune globulin, obtained from the blood of previously affected but otherwise healthy people, and waited. His confidence in recovery began to wane. He stopped eating. Soft-cop sympathy with encouragement to eat fell on stony ground. I tried the hard-cop method. He responded. He ate. He survived. It was a telling moment. He had shown vulnerability but in the end great determination and resolve to get better.

We both knew each other better after that moment and both we and Nicola recognised it.

Years later Sam spoke at various functions giving a patient's perspective of having a lung transplant. His talks were amusing, honest, personal and accurate. If he had chosen to ignore those discussions during his assessment on how hard it would be, his experience with CMV had certainly changed this view. His optimism that the future would be bright and his steely resolve offered substantial help to get him through, and he spoke eloquently of such matters.

We had many conversations during his recovery. I believe we developed a greater mutual respect as well as a better understanding. I liked him.

The Great Years, 1991–2007

'Oh, but it's magic, it's the best years of our lives.'
– Steve Harley

After recovery Sam enjoyed many years of high quality life. He returned to climbing mountains, fathered and raised a beloved family and generally returned to a normal lifestyle. Not a bad result for an experimental procedure. His joy of life regained shone through and he had fully repaid the wishes of his donor and the donor family, whose brave decision had made it all possible. Success had risen from tragedy like a phoenix from the ashes.

'Come up and see me, make me smile.
Do what you want, running wild.'
– Steve Harley

His visits to Newcastle for review became less and less frequent. They became keenly anticipated by me. These were enjoyable encounters. Conversations began discussing his health but soon expanded into mountains, whisky, the general futility of physicians and merit awards. Oh, and yes, politics!

He always managed to tease me by some of his comments, and despite my intention not to take the bait I invariably did. I would then experience that aquiline gaze and his smile. He was a neurosurgeon and me a mere physician. I could tell he liked me. I liked him. It was a good feeling.

As the years passed by he began to develop some of the inevitable consequences of long-term immunosuppression and the ageing graft. These included hypertension, skin cancers particularly on the sun-exposed surfaces ('What about the floppy hat, Sam?'), recurrent infections, a pneumothorax (air trapped between the lung and the chest wall) and 'lung allograft dysfunction', a slow but steady restriction in breathing due to a narrowing of small airway passages in the transplanted lung.

During the early stages of graft functional loss he continued with outdoor pursuits, albeit recognising his exercise tolerance was deteriorating and was limiting his abilities, leading to a gentle sense of frustration.

It was an episode of serious fungal infection in the lungs, by a mould called aspergillus, that constituted a watershed event, such that after his apparent physical recovery he was left somewhat more breathless than was ideal; but nevertheless his quality of life remained good and his spirit undiminished.

I continued to look forward to consultations. I liked him.

The Great Venture: Lung Transplantation

The Steady Years, 2007–2013

'Are you reelin' in the years, stowin' away the time?'
– Steely Dan

The medical knowledge base that underpinned success following lung transplantation was growing, particularly in respect of controlling lung infections and chronic allograft dysfunction. Sam responded to these therapies, and though his lung function did not fully recover, it stabilised and he enjoyed a further five years of productive and good-quality life. He was always in great demand to attend functions and often to speak.

2013–2014

'Not fade away.' – The Rolling Stones

Our ability to control chronic allograft dysfunction and prevent infections inevitably began to become less effective, and Sam began to be plagued by a series of recurrent bacterial infections. His exercise tolerance fell and his quality of life became frustratingly poor as far as he was concerned. He took the view that he had fully enjoyed an extended life following his transplantation, had raised a wonderful family and did not want to fade away. We shared a number of phone calls. He wanted some straight answers to questions and he knew I would give them.

When admitted in summer 2014 to the Intensive Care Unit in Glasgow with a severe pneumonia, he instructed the intensivist that he did not want to be intubated despite his worsening clinical status.

He did not fade away. Death was quick. I was saddened but understood and of course respected his decision.

Death always stimulates a period of reflection. I had learned much from him. I was astounded by his energy and love of life. I admired his principles. I respected his values. I recognised both his vulnerabilities and his strengths. He was a great role model for lung transplantation. I liked him. I always will.

Paul A. Corris

Consultant and Senior Lecturer in Respiratory Medicine, 1986–2000; Professor of Thoracic Medicine, Newcastle University, 2000 continuing.

27

Our Family

Mhairi, Heather and Fiona Galbraith, and Nicola Tennant

Our Dad: Mhairi, Heather and Fiona

Our Dad is the best. We use 'is' in the present tense because although he is gone he is still our Dad. He never really gave us any clues as to what he wanted after he was gone. His exact words were, 'I don't care, I'll be dead!' The only hint we got was when he turned up at Mhairi's medical school graduation and proudly announced that he was wearing his 'coffin suit'. Despite this, he probably spent the majority of our lives preparing us for the day we would have to live without him. He taught us the importance of working hard and stressed (repeatedly) the importance of education. He taught us resilience in tough times, how to be grateful for absolutely everything you have and how to have confidence in your own decisions. This was infuriating whenever we asked him for help to decide, because his response was always to 'do what was right'.

Although he is gone, his legacy lives on every day in the people that knew him. Dad had a huge influence on everyone in his life, and every day when we self-correct our grammar, open a text book or hear a terrible joke, we remember him. There is such a huge part of him in each of us and we are so lucky to have that.

Everything we have read about him has been very touching and suggests he was the kind of man who was good at everything he did . . . This was not the case. He played golf, at which he was terrible; he played the violin, at which he was even worse; and, in recent years, he liked to go mushroom hunting – we were never really sure whether he was any good at this or not.

Our family also has some painful memories of the time he tried to learn Spanish. Having already been told, when speaking French to someone in France, 'I'm sorry I only speak French', his Spanish hit a peak at a championship golf course, La Finca. He tried to order plates of chips, but accidently requested bananas, which were served to us on a plate by the bemused waiters. His parking skills were also questionable, but they vastly improved after he crashed into a neighbour's car who just happened to be a driving instructor, and who then gave him some lessons on parallel parking.

Another thing he enjoyed was encouraging mischief in people. He shared his trick of sticking chewing gum in keyholes with our young friend Jimmy. Later that day we listened in horror to Jimmy's dad, who told us how Jimmy had picked up a piece of chewing gum from the pavement, chewed it and then stuffed it into the keyhole in their front door.

You may have noticed that among (Dad always corrected people when they used 'between' wrongly) our Mum and the three of us, our Dad spent his family life surrounded by women. He used to say it was 'God getting back at him'. He would enjoy the wee chats he had with many of the boys in our neighbourhood, including our friend Ciaran who used to talk to him about his love of football. In recent years he enjoyed 'man chats' with Mhairi's boyfriend, Chris, relieved finally to have a man around the house. Despite what he would have you believe, Dad was a feminist at heart and had been known to let it slip that he was very proud of our independence and feminist values. This is something that the so-called 'wifies' in the Labour Party will be pleased to hear.

We don't think it mattered to Dad that we were girls. He was very busy with his work but somehow he still managed to be one of the few dads at every ballet show, every hockey game, every violin recital, every parents' night and every prize-giving. He found the time to help us with our homework and teach us how to ride our bikes. Every week we impatiently awaited Tuesday night, when Mum would go out to play badminton and Dad would lead household rebellion in the form of a 'Coke party' for the four of us. A whisky glass full of Coke and a Kit-Kat finger each was had and we could have sworn our Mum never found out! (In later years we discovered that our skills of deception had not been as good as we thought.)

During the time we spent at our chalet in Strachur, he would teach us all the things he used to do as a 'wee boy'. He taught us how to look for crabs on the beach, how to repair bicycle punctures, change car tyres, put up shelves and he would endeavour to play football with us on the grass, even though it wasn't easy for him. Come rain, shine or midges, he would brave all weathers to barbecue sausages and spare ribs with us.

Dad loved the outdoors. On our camping trips he showed us how to pitch a tent, make a fire and cook haggis, beans and tatties on the Trangia, using the salt water from the sea to cook the potatoes. In his last summer Fiona proudly sent him pictures of the fire she had built on the beach when she was camping in the Western Isles. After dinner, we'd sit around the fire toasting marshmallows, listening to his stories about his time as a Boy Scout and mountaineer, trying not to notice the midges eating us alive! Although he was no longer able to climb, he still shared his love of the mountains by taking us walking to some of his favourite places, including the Cairngorms and Duncryne Hill.

We never knew our Dad as a surgeon, although he often told us, 'Once a doctor, always a doctor.' We do, however, remember him as a politician. We have fond memories of the days of campaigning, driving through Kirkintilloch in the Butlers' Land Rover playing 'Things can only get better' out of the megaphone.

Whenever anyone asked what he'd been up to recently, his response was always the same: 'Fighting disease and ignorance single-handedly.'

When Dad retired from politics in 2001, he took over all the cooking in our house. He produced dishes such as crayfish tails and squid, which did not go down well with us, especially after Mhairi had been left traumatised as a three-year-old when he threw a langoustine into her paddling pool. Over time he homed in on our tastes and became very proud of his skills as a chef, teaching anyone who would listen the correct way to chop up an onion. He never quite got the idea of the weekly shop however; having received 36 litres of orange juice from his first online order he then decided he liked to visit the supermarket daily to hand-pick the ingredients for our dinner that night.

Dad was many different things to many different people: a doctor, a politician, a patient, a friend, a brother. His work was very important to him and he achieved much success as a neurosurgeon and latterly as a politician, but there is no doubt in our minds that to him, his most important role was as a husband and a father. He always said his goal was to send us off to university with a good set of teeth and a driving licence; after that his job would be done.

Dad would have done anything for us and he proved this on many occasions, most recently when he flew to London and back in a morning to deliver Heather's passport so we could go to Disneyland. He always taught us that family is the most important thing in life, and one of his most prized possessions was a bed built for him by his father and his two brothers. He often recounted how our granddad and uncles had seen him sleeping on a mattress on the floor when he first started working as a junior doctor. They collected driftwood from the beach and fallen trees and made a spectacular double bed, our granddad being a joiner. This bed is still going strong many years later in our house in Glasgow.

Although he was taken from us far too soon, we are grateful for the time we had together. We understand that we might have grown up without him and appreciate every lesson we learned and every moment we shared. Many might ask what it was that made his transplant quite so successful, but his answer was always very clear: he said it was 'a life of high moral rectitude, and being nice to women.'

We will miss him so much.

Sam: Nicola

> Had we never lov'd sae kindly,
> Had we never lov'd sae blindly,
> Never met – or never parted –
> We had ne'er been broken-hearted.

Sam, having inscribed this verse from 'Ae Fond Kiss' in my treasured French dictionary, drove me to the airport, bought me a double whisky and I left for Switzerland. I had always planned to travel and to work abroad; I hadn't 'planned' on Sam, however, and as we parted, no promises made, I considered that our time together may have come to an end.

We met in 1979, in the Institute of Neurological Sciences at the Southern General Hospital, Glasgow. The Institute hill-walking club introduced me to the Scottish mountains and to Sam. Immediately it was clear that he was different, the formalities of the hospital hierarchy were not for him, he was known to everyone just as 'Sam' – and there was more than a hint of a serious sense of fun. We spent the following two years walking, climbing and camping in Glen Coe, Sutherland, Skye, Fort William and on the 'Ben', not forgetting the many Friday evenings in the Aragon bar in Byres Road.

When I met Sam he lived a Spartan life, often sleeping on the hard floor in preference to his soft warm bed in order to toughen himself up for 'the mountains'. He had little regard for material goods, had few casual clothes and was instantly recognisable in his deerstalker hat and elbow-less tweed jacket. He paid little attention to the mundane activities of daily life, like washing dishes, for example. One day his sister, Ailsa, found a mouldy cup and assumed he must be carrying out an experiment! His flat was furnished with a couple of mugs, paper plates, plastic knives and forks, one sofa, a bust of Lenin and an empty fridge – empty apart from the Beluga caviar donated by a visiting registrar. His pride and joy, other than his climbing and camping equipment, was his vast collection of books: philosophical (at least four copies of Plato's *Republic*), political and medical. Novels and fiction he thought too frivolous.

Sandy, his good friend and comrade, lived in the flat above: an erudite pathologist with a similar philosophy of life to Sam's and equally Spartan in his existence. They had both climbed with the Glasgow University Mountaineering (GUM) Club, later to become 'The Desperados'. Sam, Sandy and I spent many great days, evenings and Hogmanays up North with them; camping, walking, climbing and 'Stripping the Willow' in the snow as Chris the fiddler rattled off 'Caddam Woods'! The 'purvey' was legendary, from Yan's quails' eggs and beautifully, but extremely slowly, roasted goose (often served after midnight) to Sandy's slices of borsch soup (which eventually diluted actually to become soup). Stories of previous exploits and debates were always a regular feature, as was Sandy reading *Das Kapital* in German. Many songs, including the Scottish Mountaineering Club's anthem 'Oh, My Big Hobnailers' to the tune of 'Oh, Dem Golden Slippers', were sung and ridiculous games played.

Each summer, Sam and Sandy took off for the Alps in Sandy's car, a Citroen 2CV or as Sam called it, the 'sewing machine'.

With it packed full of climbing gear and camping equipment, and with little room for personal niceties such as clean underwear, they set off. After a few circuits of the Boulevard Périphérique in the environs of Paris they arrived in Chamonix, where they climbed and read for a month. In 1986, he and Sandy set off as part of an expedition to the Himalayas. The plan was to conquer an unclimbed peak, which in the event of a successful ascent was to be named 'Partickhill'. It was a dreadful year in the Himalayas, and they became stranded in storms and drifting snow. They were well above base-camp and had to dig and climb their way out and down the mountain, snow storms not abating. They were lucky to survive.

During winter seasons in the Cairngorms with the 'Aragon' team of Hamiltons, Burnses, Bradleys and Sandy, Sam and Sandy climbed and others skied. With the introduction of 'future wives', except in Sandy's case, Sam's resolve weakened. He eventually came over to the dark side and learned to ski, becoming one of those 'plankers' he loved to abuse (Harry's hairy wellies always fair game). We then spent some wonderful times ski mountaineering with our 'peau de phoque' and non-waisted, impossible-to-turn skis. We even cross-country skied in Glasgow one snowy winter's night, down Gardner Street to Dumbarton Road and along to the Aragon!

Sam did visit Switzerland, and when I left, travelling still, we continued with a distant relationship across several continents. Having worked and toured in Australia, travelled in China, Thailand, Malaysia, Indonesia and India, I moved to New Brunswick, Canada, in 1984. Sam was then Visiting Professor at Dartmouth College in New Hampshire. We met and skied in Killington, Vermont; we ate lobster in Maine and visited Montreal and Quebec. Our favourite haunt was 'Molly's Balloon' in Hanover, New Hampshire, where we would meet Quentin, a colleague of Sam's at Dartmouth, and his wife Barbara Ann.

They later visited us in Glasgow, as did Sam's good friends Gary and Kathy from Texas. Sam returned to Glasgow and I remained in Canada. I loved Canada and the outdoor lifestyle, but I was drawn back to Scotland and returned later that year.

Sam had always been politically active and was then a member of the, at times beleaguered, Partick Anderston branch of the Labour Party. He had campaigned in the 1982 Hillhead (Roy Jenkins) by-election, championed the cause of health workers and was part of the Medical Aid for Nicaragua Campaign. In a similar vein to Brian Wilson's story about Julie Christie ('What do you do yourself, Julia?') Sam, at a small fundraising gathering on the south side of Glasgow, was heard to ask David Hayman if 'he got much work?'!

He was speaking at Party meetings all over Scotland and was adopted as the Labour Party candidate for Strathkelvin and Bearsden in 1986. It was an amazing campaign, with the hub of the Bearsden operation being in the Butlers' house. Grahame Smith was Sam's election agent and Hilda went on to become Sam's much tried and tested secretary. The campaign culminated at the count, the excitement palpable, as Sam took Strathkelvin and Bearsden. However opposition, not government, was looming.

We were married in Kingussie in 1987, with Harry, Senga and eight-month-old Maria as our witnesses. We had planned to live there, somewhat optimistically as Sam had been diagnosed with the lung condition fibrosing alveolitis. Although he was then still well, even with the sleeper link between Inverness and London it would have been difficult. It was a horrific transition to Westminster for many of the new MPs. There was nowhere to stay; Sam was admitted to the Chelsea and Westminster hospital with a viral infection primarily because he was 'homeless' in London. However, it all started to look up, or so I thought, when he and Brian found a flat in Bethnal Green. It was only when I visited I realised that Sam was sleeping on a mattress of newspapers on the floor! Life in London could only get better.

Sam was instrumental in his sister Katherine's diagnosis of fibrosing alveolitis, for which she had a heart and lung transplant at Papworth Hospital in 1989. By then, I was pregnant with Mhairi and it became apparent that Sam's condition was following the same course. Mhairi was a few weeks old when we had our first visit to the Freeman Hospital in Newcastle. He was assessed for a single lung transplant and listed. Sam continued to deteriorate, he was admitted to the Western Infirmary in December 1989 and timeously he received his transplant on 5 January 1990 in Newcastle. Our time at the Freeman was fraught; there was initial elation at being there, the transplant going ahead and Sam surviving. The new lung seemed to be functioning, but each morning our day and life was determined by Sam's temperature, a key rejection indicator. The nursing and medical staff were wonderful – they had the measure of Sam! There was caring, kindness, respect, honesty and much cajoling. Paul Corris's statement, 'Sam, if you don't eat you don't shit, and if you don't shit you die', is legendary within the family. Sam got the message.

The help and assistance from both our families was amazing; some of them came and stayed with me in hospital accommodation to help with the practicalities of having a four-month-old baby (babies could not visit ITU). Roderick and Lynn had driven Mhairi and me down and were an incredible support throughout. Friends visited with all manner of food to tempt Sam to eat. After a particularly tense few days I bought a bottle of Sam's favourite malt whisky, Talisker. Fortunately, a wee dram had the desired therapeutic effect; Sam's shoulders came down from being up around his ears, his 'white-knuckle' grip on the arms of the chair relaxed and calm descended upon us. After concerns about rejection and subsequent infection, we came back to Glasgow and Sam continued to improve. Tragically, his older sister Katherine had died during this time, leaving a bereft family. Sam, already grateful for his second chance, was now determined to make the most of it.

We moved to Jordanhill in 1991. At that time my mother had emergency coronary artery bypass surgery, Sam pointing out to her that she had been a hypochondriac for years, yet, when seriously ill, she neglected to mention it! When Heather was born in January 1992 and Fiona in August 1993, my parents were invaluable to us. Often, when they came to babysit, rather than go out, we would promptly go to bed and sleep!

The girls attended Jordanhill School. They all did well academically. We attended prize-giving every year until Fiona left in 6th year as School Dux. Mhairi had been School Captain, Heather Vice-Captain. We always enjoyed school music concerts with Mhairi and Heather both playing the violin and flute, Fiona the clarinet. Mhairi was leader of the band. Sam also played the violin as a boy and had taken it up again – amazing everyone and instantly impressing them when he mentioned that his teacher was in fact Nicola Benedetti's teacher! This was true; she had taught Nicola Benedetti as a youngster.

All three girls played hockey for Hillhead Hockey Club and Heather, as Captain of the School First XI in her final year, banned Sam from watching as he was regularly heard shouting 'Get intae them!' from the side-line. Despite his punishing parliamentary workload, he attended all their ballet displays at Mrs Christie's Ballet School and at Scottish Ballet, but when we attended Mhairi's ballet performance at Cambridge University, he said that would be his last; he had indeed done his bit. He regularly did the gymnastics run, watched them in competitions, attended cross-country events and took Heather to Tollcross swimming pool for 5.30 a.m. training sessions. Even in his final weeks in June, he struggled to get the train and walk to the new

Commonwealth pitch at Glasgow Green to watch Fiona play for Edinburgh University, and win the plate on Scottish Hockey cup final day.

Sam has instilled his socialist values in all the girls, taking them on the campaign trail throughout the constituency, including the leafy suburbs of Bearsden, where in their enthusiasm they even leafleted the exclusive all-male Glasgow Golf Club at Killermont! They were brought up with politicians, civil servants and the odd film crew dropping in and out of our house, and they particularly remember Donald Dewar; he was immensely tall, thin, chatty and always starving! The benefits were trips to London, seeing Westminster, staying in No. 10 when Alistair was Chancellor and also visiting the Scottish Parliament. Sam went out of his way to protect them from any fallout from his days as Health Minister, and the trials and tribulations of being Education Minister. As the SQA exam story broke in August 2000, a swift return from our summer holidays in Lewis was interspersed with several stops at phone-boxes (pre mobile phones) en route to Glasgow. It was inevitable that the girls would be affected; we were all affected.

Fortunately there were few occasions when the press (or the trappings of political life) invaded our privacy, but in 2000 as Section 28 of the Local Government Act was repealed in Scotland, the group behind a vicious campaign against the repeal was responsible for a billboard emblazoned with a huge photograph of Sam vilifying him for his stance. This appeared a few hundred yards from the girls' school and where we lived.

Despite his move to the Department of Education, his first love was health and he was resolute in his mission to improve the nation's health. He felt it was his duty as a doctor to point out to people that they were overweight, which he did with gusto! For as long as I have known Sam, obesity and smoking (teeth also featured) were top of the agenda when it came to proffering his often brutal advice. He took no prisoners, as many can testify. Those who were not obese still had to be concerned about being 'crypto-obese'.

Recently, one of Sam's Scottish Office friends, 'Luggsy', said in a lovely email that Sam had been very proud of his girls' feminism! He constantly teased and goaded them, and me in particular, into lengthy discussions/arguments about our 'loony feminist rubbish'. However, he astonished us all when, having been summoned to the girls' school, he announced to a teacher with whom Fiona had had a slightly overly heated debate that 'he was very proud of his ten-year-old daughter being aware of gender issues'! He often said that God was getting back at him by surrounding him with four women, but according to a friend of mine, who worked for the Women's Support Network, a 4:1 ratio was just about right for Sam. He did, however, have some credentials. He and Sandy campaigned relentlessly for the Scottish Mountaineering Club to admit women, which they eventually did. He was always in favour of the admission of women to the hallowed turf of the R&A in St Andrews and this, he knew, was imminent, as his great friend David Hamilton, an R&A member, had spotted 'Ladies' toilets within!

He always took great delight in shocking and irritating the girls and their friends with his lavatorial humour or terrible jokes; cries of 'DAAAD!' as he announced yet again that he was 'coughing up someone else's phlegm'. He teased incessantly! He told the girls that it is the person you are that is important and not how you look, but they quickly cottoned onto this as his excuse for him to wear the same clothes until they fell apart. They did finally realise that he genuinely didn't care what he wore or how he looked when he was seen walking round the corner to Kate and Harpreet's in his pyjamas. The girls learned with time to take what he said with a pinch of salt. As he castigated them for driving too fast they pointed out that for someone who overshot a bend and ended up in Loch Lomond in his MGB GT, this was a bit rich! He had also been stopped for speeding on the A9. When the police reminded him that the speed limit was 60 mph and not 70 mph, he announced to said police that he had been breaking the law for years!

Transport and travel seemed to be a recurring theme. When he retired from politics we went on holiday to America. As we were about to board the plane, having gone through passport control, one of the airside staff noticed that Sam's passport was out of date. He was aghast, of course; he had been travelling to Europe for months as a minister with an invalid passport. He had also, while working for the General Medical Council in Manchester, booked himself into the Hilton, only to discover on arrival that his room was in the Hilton in Manchester, New Hampshire, USA! He conceded afterwards that the fact he'd paid in US dollars might have been a clue.

Even when he was unable to climb in the mountains, he was always keen to get out of the city and up north. Sam loved his time as the locum surgeon at the Broadford Hospital in Skye and he loved few places more than the Western Isles. Before and after his transplant we had wonderful visits to Brian and Joni's in Uig. The girls loved the beaches in Lewis, particularly body-surfing at Bosta with the Wilsons and the Darlings. In Benbecula there was swimming with the Galbraith girl cousins, most memorably the time we stayed with Karen and Nairn and Sam developed pneumonia that signalled the end of his part in the family tradition of 'freezing water' swimming. Many of the girls' early years were spent at Strachur on Loch Fyne, where they swam in the loch with their cousins until literally blue with cold. The barbecue-toasted marshmallows, somehow, made it worthwhile. We enjoyed Graham and Evelyn's hospitality at Fernachan on Loch Fyne where the girls learned to fish and had great fun learning to water-ski.

The funicular at Cairngorm allowed Sam some time in the mountains. The girls and I, or Ailsa and I, would meet him at the Ptarmigan restaurant when we had been either skiing or walking. He kept up his interest in flora and fauna, and the girls have endured many tutorials on sphagnum moss and the difference between bracken and fern. He became an avid mycologist, identifying and describing the many, many types of mushrooms in Latin to us all. Always striving to be in the outdoors, Sam took up golf, playing with his brother Roderick at the municipal course he called 'Royal Knightswood', and latterly with his good friends Harpreet and Ray at Ross Priory. Although his delight in taking alfresco pees was well known, he finally realised that the middle of the fairway on a golf course (particularly the 4th at Milngavie) was not really acceptable.

As time marched on, life became more challenging from a health perspective. Socialising was always difficult for Sam despite his ability to be the life and soul of the party; he found standing or even sitting at a table for dinner exhausting. At family gatherings, unless engaged in some semantic debate about the difference between 'shall' and 'will', he would often slope off for a snooze. We had good philosophical and political debates as the girls got older, and many a lively evening was had debating at home, and at friends' houses. The Independence Referendum, as the debate gained momentum, was the last.

Sam continued to attend appointments in Newcastle, which were approached with apprehension but also with a degree of pleasure at seeing the team and getting the latest gossip. He stayed with his friend Alistair, a neurosurgeon, where he enjoyed his 'veggie scran' and more gossip. In Glasgow he attended pulmonary rehab classes and, although he had my physiotherapy colleagues tearing their hair out, he really did get the importance of physical activity. In the winter he regularly went to our local shopping centre, where it was warm, to walk up and down the stairs in a bid to increase his exercise tolerance. We had a number of serious health scares over the years, many with hospital admissions, which was possibly why the final one came as such a shock to us all. We began to think he was invincible.

Summer 2014 was a wonderful summer for Sam. He, Ailsa and I swam in the River Truim, the weather being uncharacteristically hot. This was the first time Sam had been swimming outdoors for years. We also walked to the River Calder in the Monadhliaths where, half an hour off the beaten track and not another soul in sight, a couple appeared, only to say: 'Aren't you Sam Galbraith?'! He continued to be recognised wherever he went.

He once thought he would never see Mhairi grow up, but not only has he seen one daughter into her adult life, he has seen three. He was incredibly proud of Mhairi going to Cambridge and becoming a doctor; he also knew Chris, now her husband, and would have been delighted, not at the thought of a wedding, but at the prospect of Chris as his son-in-law. He saw Heather graduate with her law degree from Edinburgh University in July 2014 and would be both proud and envious of her studying Human Rights at Columbia University in New York. Fiona had completed three of her five years in chemical engineering at Edinburgh University, and he greatly approved of her two summers' coaching tennis and hockey in Massachusetts.

Sam has had a great influence on us all, but especially the girls, showing them it is important to make the most of what you have and never to look back at what might have been. They saw first-hand his indomitable, amazing spirit.

It was fitting that at the end Mhairi came up from London as a junior doctor and, with her sisters in America, she took charge. She was there at the beginning of his transplant journey and at the end. In conjunction with the ITU staff she helped manage it as Sam wished.

The girls know how lucky they have been to have him as their Dad for the time that they did, and they adored him as he did them. We miss him every day and will miss him always.

Ae fond kiss, and then we sever.
Ae farewell, alas, for ever.

Mhairi Galbraith

Graduate in Medicine, University of Cambridge, 2013; Registrar in Public Health, East of England.

Heather Galbraith

Graduate in Law, University of Edinburgh, 2014; Postgraduate Student of Human Rights, Columbia University, New York.

Fiona Galbraith

Final Year Undergraduate Student in Chemical Engineering, University of Edinburgh.

Nicola Tennant

Physiotherapy Advanced Practitioner in Clinical Gait Analysis, Specialist Children's Services, Greater Glasgow and Clyde.

28

Some Speeches and Writings

Maiden Speech, Westminster
House of Commons

23 October 1987
[Extract from the Official Report]

POLITICS IS HEALTH
Speech by SAM GALBRAITH, M.P.

Mr Sam Galbraith (Strathkelvin and Bearsden): I congratulate
the hon. Member for Norfolk, South-West (Mrs Shephard) on
her excellent maiden speech. I was particularly impressed by her
description of her constituency. It is obviously a beautiful place
to live and work. I took to heart her description of the problems
in the delivery of health care over such a wide area. Those problems are, indeed, very difficult to solve and I am only too well
aware of them in an area such as the Highlands and Islands. It is
a matter to which we should direct our attention. I am sure that
the House is grateful to the hon. Lady for her remarks, which
were delivered in an excellent and articulate manner.

I pay tribute to my predecessor, Mr Michael Hirst. Michael
and I were at university together and I well remember him from
the debating chambers of Glasgow University Union, where he
polished his skills in preparation for the day when he would be
a Member of Parliament. I understand that he used those skills
highly effectively in this Chamber. My constituents have mentioned my predecessor a number of times and remarked on what
an excellent constituency Member he was. It is clear from what

they say that he spared no effort to look after them and deal with their problems. I trust that I will be able to do even better than he did. I should like to thank him on behalf of my constituents for the work that he has done in the past.

I am glad to be able to make my maiden speech in this debate on health, for a number of reasons. Health is of particular importance to my constituents. Bearsden is often described in our national dailies as a leafy suburb. That part of Strathkelvin is made up of Bishopbriggs, Kirkintilloch and the villages of Lennoxtown and Torrance and lies beneath the Campsie hills and along the Kelvin river. My constituency has a small industrial base of under 2,000 jobs. The largest single employer is the Health Service. That is why health is of particular importance to my constituency.

I am also pleased to be able to speak in a debate on health because I have been employed in that sector for many years. I must warn the House to be wary of so-called experts such as myself and my large hon. Friend the Member for Kirkcaldy (Dr Moonie). People such as he and I tend to peddle our prejudices and ride our hobbyhorses. My hobbyhorse is the acute sector, its inadequate provision and its inefficient method of delivering care. That is a subject to which I shall return in the ensuing months.

But to avoid peddling prejudices, I shall talk about the promotion of health. It is a subject that is not often dealt with by doctors in the acute sector. Doctors in the acute sector are concerned with the provision of services for the treatment of disease, not specifically the promotion of health, and there is an important difference. The treatment of disease is a proper and excellent end, but it is not the same as the promotion of health. If my specialty were to disappear overnight – let us not pretend that that will happen – and there were no neurosurgeons tomorrow, there would be no significant effect on the nation's health, although a significant effect on suffering.

The promotion of health is a separate subject. It is not necessarily about the acute sector, although that is an important aspect, or about the regular checkups advertised by private organisations offering services at highly inflated prices. In such cases, a number of investigations are carried out, blood pressure is checked, chest X-rays performed and various nondescript tests of no value performed. Promotion of health is not about measuring the serum cholesterol. It is about preventing it from going up – an important point to consider.

We must grasp the fact that the promotion of health is a political issue. I am disappointed that only the junior Health Minister – the hon. Member for Derbyshire, South (Mrs Currie) – is present and that the Secretary of State for Employment, the Minister of Agriculture, Fisheries and Food, and the Chancellor of the Exchequer are not here. Every one of them should be here, because they are more important in promoting health than anyone else.

When I started medicine, rheumatic fever was a common disease, causing abnormalities and valvular disease of the heart. Nowadays, a medical student does not have to waste time listening for opening snaps and mitral stenosis. Perhaps my hon. Friend the Member for Kirkcaldy will tell me about that later, because I have forgotten.

When I was a medical student, one could not even mention tuberculosis because it was such a terrible disease. In the town in which I was brought up, we all had relatives who had died of that disease. Rheumatic fever has disappeared and tuberculosis has become a minor disease. This happened not because of doctors, streptomycin or penicillin but because political activity has changed our social structure and social environment. The change occurred in my town because the Labour-controlled local authority gave everyone a decent house. There were school meals, good education and mass campaigns. They are important in the promotion of health. It is not necessarily a matter of doctors treating disease.

The promotion of health is changing slightly. We now talk about changing lifestyles. I am pleased that the Under-Secretary of State talked about footballers taking alcohol. That is a political issue which requires political action. The hon. Lady cannot hedge away by saying that she wants to get us all to co-operate, although that is important. But she will have to take political initiatives.

The Under-Secretary of State would like us to co-operate and encourage people. One should not start in the way the hon. Lady did when she was appointed junior Minister and blame everyone, saying, 'It is all your fault. It is a matter of what you eat. If you did not eat this food, you would not get this disease.' She spoke as though she had just discovered some new great philosophy on health, whereas we had been campaigning for changes for many years. To get people to co-operate, we should not blame them. We should take them along with our ideas and make facilities available. I welcome the Heartbeat award, which is a useful innovation. Perhaps the Under-Secretary of State will get the Under-Secretary of State for Scotland – the hon. Member for Stirling (Mr Forsyth) – who has responsibility for health in Scotland, to look at what is happening in some hospitals, particularly the one in which I worked, which had such facilities.

It was particularly noticeable that the Under-Secretary of State for Health and Social Security did not mention unemployment in connection with health. I can well understand why. There is no question but that there is a relationship between unemployment and health. All the evidence suggests that there is. What is that relationship? Is it spurious? Is it causal and, if so, in what way? Does unemployment cause ill health or does ill health cause unemployment? Some publications show that unemployment clearly causes ill health, especially in terms of mental health. A Sheffield study, which was reported in *Psychological Medicine* in 1982, investigated two groups of school leavers. Those who became unemployed showed a far greater incidence of mental disorders than the employed, whereas the incidence of mental disorders was the same for both groups when at school. That clearly showed a causal relationship between ill health and unemployment.

There is a causal relationship between unemployment and physical ill health. A 1984 *Lancet* publication of an article by Mosner *et al*, using information from the Office of Population Censuses and Surveys, showed that in cohorts people who became unemployed had higher standard mortality ratios than those who did not – a ratio of 136. The survey showed that unemployment caused early deaths. It showed that there was no significant increase in the first five years, which is what one would have expected. The survey showed that the wives of the men who became unemployed had higher standard mortality ratios than the wives of employed men, which is what one would expect if unemployment causes ill health.

We can no longer dodge the issue by saying that the evidence is inconclusive. There is a clear causal relationship between unemployment and ill health. Unemployment causes ill health. This requires political solutions. The promotion of health is a political issue which requires political action by every Department. No Department can shrink from this. Together they can promote health, add years to people's lives and life to those extra years. I call upon the Government to take this action.

'Talking to Patients – The Golden Rules'

Glasgow Herald, 22 January 1991

I was a young doctor, just out of medical school. I still believed what my elders told me. We were doing the morning ward round, and were just leaving the patient with cancer when he called us back. He had recently undergone major surgery.

'Tell me, doc,' he said, 'have I got cancer?'

'Not at all, my good man,' replied the consultant, 'you will live to be 100.' We moved on.

The patient was not convinced. An intelligent man in his 60s, he wanted to be informed, not patronised. Everything was wrong. There had to be a better way.

As young doctors we were brought up to deceive, never to tell the truth when the news was bad. The word 'cancer' was forbidden. Rather we talked of 'neoplasia' and 'mitotic figures'. Tuberculosis was still taboo. The euphemism used was 'Koch's disease'. Yes, there had to be a better way when talking to patients, especially if the news was bad.

A lot of it cannot be taught. You either have it or you do not. Being good with people and able to relate to their experiences helps. A sense of one's own mortality is also helpful. In the end, however, you have to work out most of it for yourself.

But, as young struggling doctors, some reference points would have been helpful, some general principles useful. So here are mine, my three golden rules and three practical guidelines for communicating with patients. They have been worked out over the years with a lot of help from my friends and former colleagues. They refer to doctors but apply equally well to all those others who talk to patients, indeed more often and sometimes better than doctors.

'**Never lie to the patient.**' If you stick to this rule, there will be few mistakes. I never, ever regretted telling anyone the truth about cancer or other fatal diseases. I have regretted not telling them.

I still remember a patient with whom I had been less than candid. She found out the truth; I eventually told her. She never trusted me again. I looked after her for ten years before she died, but never regained her confidence. Each time we spoke, I could see her questioning and wondering if I was telling the truth. I felt uneasy in her company. I had betrayed her. Never again.

Trust is the basis of the doctor/patient relationship. Lacking knowledge the patient is vulnerable and trust is essential. Without it, the relationship is nothing and so is the care. In any event, the patient is entitled to the truth.

My second rule is, '**Never force information on the patient.**' I take it as accepted that everyone is entitled, as soon as possible, to the fullest information within the limits of knowledge and comprehension. But there are a few who just do not want to know and we have no right to force bad news upon them.

When to hold back is, I am afraid, one of these things that cannot be taught. It can only come from experience. After a time, however, it is possible to recognise the patient who simply just does not want to know.

The opening gambit is never, 'Sorry, you've got cancer.' Rather the subject is slowly introduced and those who don't want to know call a halt early on. Patients have all sorts of ways of signalling. You then have a second go and once again the shutters come up. It is time to stop. Deep down, the patient knows what's wrong but does not want formally to acknowledge it. In this way they keep their hope.

This takes me to my third and final rule, '**Never leave the patient without hope.**' It does not involve lying, which would break the first and most important rule. Nor does it involve being unrealistic. But it does mean putting particular weight on the rare or unexpected occurrence.

The outcome from cancer may be bad, but there are always those who do surprisingly well. You emphasise this to the patient. You know and they know the chances of them personally doing as well are small. But there is a chance, and this is what gives them hope.

Realistically, they accept the worst and are prepared for it, all the time sustained by the knowledge that there might be a chance. No hope, no future. No person is entitled to remove this from the patient.

Rules alone, however, are insufficient. Patients are people with complex responses and needs. When applying rules, attitudes and behaviour are just as important. Again, there are three important points.

'**Look the patient straight in the eye.**' If not, they wonder what you are hiding. Why is the doctor so shifty? What's really wrong with me? When you look them straight in the eye, they know it's the truth.

'**Take plenty of time with the patient.**' The outpatient clinic is rarely the place to reveal shattering news. Many times I would admit the patient on the pretext of further investigation, but really with the intention of slowly introducing the true magnitude of their illness.

A chair is essential. As you sit down, the patient knows they have your time and undivided attention. Standing signals that you are in a hurry, and even worse is the nervous shuffling towards the door. A person's life is about to be shattered, sitting down isn't too much.

'**Never patronise the patient.**' As doctors we often talk to patients as if they were babies. I used to be infuriated by the snotty-nosed young doctor, just out of medical school, who spoke to patients as if they were in rompers. Often these patients had fought in one if not two world wars, been through a recession and brought up large families. In their presence, the young doctor should have been respectful, if not somewhat awed. Never patronise.

In the same vein, doctors must never allow their moral and social prejudices to masquerade as medical judgements or determine behaviour. Everyone, no matter their colour, sex or political class, has emotions, feels the pain of death and the loss of a loved one. We all bleed. In sickness, we are all equal and should be treated as such.

Rules and practical tips are aids, not absolutes. They do not and can never account for every situation that will arise. The human condition is too varied and rich for this ever to be possible. But rules can help. Medicine is, after all, about human beings, not high-tech machines. Talking to computers is easy. Talking to people is more difficult.

'The Art of Moving Mountains'

Scotsman, Friday 3 January 1992

Many years ago Sam Galbraith was enchanted by the peaks of Skye. He recently returned to find he was still under the island's spell.

We crossed the ferry at Kyle of Lochalsh and sped onwards. Through Broadford, past Luib and up the hill, skirting the Red Cuillins. Coming down the other side, the pulse quickened. Would it be the same? After a few years away, was I living with memories or was there still something special?

With Sconser and the Raasay Ferry behind us, we turned the corner and there they were, Sgurr nan Gillean, Am-Bhaister and the Tooth – the Cuillins in all their majesty and wonder. It was the magic of Skye.

My wife and I had last visited Skye two years previously for what I thought was my last trip. I had held up my daughter of a few weeks to the mountains. The peaks and the future were hers. But we were all back. I quickly pulled into the car park at the Sligachan Hotel, opened the door and got out. I was standing on the hallowed ground once more.

For climbers, Skye is a special place. We all have our preferences, usually depending on where we live – Glencoe, Ben Nevis, Lochnagar, Cairngorms and the Northern Highlands. But for everyone, Skye is different. Its memories linger on.

The excitement of climbing in Skye would start on the Thursday night. Everything had to be prepared for a quick getaway on Friday after work. As always, the anticipation was part of the pleasure. Come 5 o'clock on the Friday, all were assembled, the car slammed into gear and the race was on to reach the Sligachan Hotel before it closed at 10 o'clock.

It was possible to reach Kyle of Lochalsh in three and a half hours, but you had to drive up Loch Lomondside at 80 miles an hour in third gear on the wrong side of the road. But we were young then and life was lived to the full.

The first crisis of the weekend would come at Kintail Lodge. Fifteen minutes from the ferry, we had to decide if we would still reach Sligachan on time, or whether refreshments should be partaken in Kintail. Funny how the driver always thought we should push on!

The second crisis would come at the ferry. Here lay the key to the world record time between Glasgow and Sligachan. Miss a ferry and arrival at Sligachan before last orders was in doubt. Ah, the benefits now of 'Clayson' and the late opening.

Driving up the road, even at speed, we absorbed the scenery in all its splendour – Glencoe, Ben Nevis, Invergarry, Glenshiel, Eilean Donan Castle, and the Kyles themselves. It was part of the spell. We were never bored.

Despite the short trip, you felt on crossing the ferry and reaching Kyleakin that you had travelled a huge distance in mind and attitude.

You were on an island, separated from the mainland with all its troubles. You had that sense of detachment – one of the attractions of climbing – even without climbing. Islands and mountains are together a potent and tangible combination of happiness and fulfilment. I hope the bridge doesn't spoil it.

In Sligachan you can still feel the presence of the climbing greats. The faded and battered old pictures in the dirty unhygienic bar added to their presence. Alas, it has now gone, replaced by a clinical barn with the atmosphere of a railway cafeteria. Is it progress, or am I just becoming old and conservative?

No more wild camping either. It was never great around the Sligachan Burn, with the ground being either too hard to get the pegs in, or too bumpy to sleep. But herded into official sites with hot and cold running water is not what the adventure is about. Again, I suppose it is the inevitable progress of time, but I don't have to like it, or approve.

But change cannot remove from the mountains the presence and atmosphere of the giants, 'Mallory Slab and Groove', 'Collie's Route' to the Cioch – you can almost feel the great men.

And what of 'Naismith's Route' on the Bhaister Tooth? I will never forget the sickening feeling in my stomach as I looked out over the ledge at what was supposed to be a 'Diff'. The instant exposure and depth made the route look impossible. It isn't. The exposure is there, the sense of separation is there. Fortunately so are the holds.

Then there is the Cuillin Ridge, the ultimate for all climbers. Its many miles, and many peaks traversed in a day of walking, scrambling and rock climbing is a good test of the mountaineer's ability.

With two medical colleagues, Ewan Macdonald and Sandy Reid, I had been trying for a number of years to traverse the Ridge. As we had climbed together for many years, we wanted to do the Ridge together. But the weather was never right. Our ways would soon separate so we had to move quickly.

As always we chose September when the midges are fewer and the tourists dwindling.

Leaving on the Friday evening, Macdonald and I were exhausted. Young doctors, we had been up all of the previous night. Reid, the pathologist, had no such problem.

As we sped up through Invergarry and down Glenshiel the rain battered on the windscreen. The prospects were not good, but we hadn't bothered about the weather forecast, our excuse being that in these days they were unreliable.

In reality, of course, with the arrogance of our youth, we thought ourselves immune to the laws of nature and, in any event, could handle anything.

Rather than camp at Sligachan, we went on to Glenbrittle – our first mistake. We thought we could get an early start and could save time by camping as near the beginning of the Ridge as possible.

We put our tent up about midnight and considered setting off. We should have. But we were so exhausted with our previous sleepless night that we decided to grab two hours before setting off.

It was 4 o'clock when we awoke. We were already behind schedule. The first stage from Garsbheinn went easily, as did the 'Thearlach-Dubh Gap', 'King's Chimney' and the Inaccessible Pinnacle. The hard climbing was behind us, but the bad weather was in front.

The mist came down and it started raining. At first we were relieved because our water had already run out, but the rain continued and the mist got lower. The climbing from then on is relatively easy, but there is a considerable amount of exposed scrambling, which in the rain is more difficult.

No time to hold back and no time for precautions. We had to crack on and do everything solo. Eventually we were over Am-Bhaister, round the Gendarme, and finally stood on the summit of Sgurr nan Gillean.

The rain could not dampen our spirits. Macdonald, Reid and I would soon be going our separate ways, but for now we shared the mountains.

There was still no time to wait around. We had to try and get back to the hotel before the bar closed in order to get a lift for Glenbrittle. In these days the pubs closed at 10, so we cracked on.

The slog-out was interminable. Lamps were taken out and the inevitable accepted, we would not make it to the hotel in time. We arrived at the road, wet, cold and tired. How we wished we had pitched our tents in Sligachan.

Sandy eventually hitched a lift from the barman who took him to Carbost, his blood alcohol (the barman's, not Sandy's) probably at an unrecordable level.

After standing in the cold at the road end for an hour and a half, Sandy stopped the first car returning from the ceilidh in Portree. It took him on to Glenbrittle where he picked up our car. We were glad to see him return. It was after 3 a.m. when we reached our tent.

We rose in the morning still exhausted, but still elated. The mountains, which were clear of mist, looked even grander. All around the place seemed to ooze a mixture of beauty, majesty and contentment.

This trip I was merely passing through on my way to a family holiday in the outer isles. And yet I still had the same great feelings. Perhaps next time a climb. But for now I was satisfied. I had stood once again on the island and it had not let me down.

'William Hutchison Murray: Larger-than-Life Hero of the Mountains'

West Highland Free Press, Friday 26 April 1996

Labour MP Sam Galbraith, a keen climber and hillwalker, pays a personal tribute to a Scottish mountaineering giant.

William Hutchison Murray died recently at the age of 83. He was a Scottish mountaineering giant. Along with Mackenzie, Dunn and MacAlpine, he became a larger-than-life hero and dominated the Scottish climbing scene before the War.

I met Bill Murray briefly on only a few occasions. And yet, like many mountaineers, I felt I knew him well. This was because of his books.

Mountaineering in Scotland is one of the finest climbing books ever written. I have read it three times completely and on many, many other occasions, dipped in to read a chapter. It is sheer joy. The style may be over-elaborate, but Murray undoubtedly captures within this book what mountaineering is all about.

You can enjoy the great pleasures of the scenery and the climb and at the same time experience the sweating palms, as he describes his epics on Crowberry Ridge on the Buachaille Etive Mor, Deep-Cut Chimney on Stob Coire nam Beith, and the Crack of Doom in Skye – individually, each one of them a story in its own right, and all described in Murray's splendid narrative.

The story of the book is itself classic Murray. In 1942, he was captured in North Africa and spent the next few years in prisoner-of-war camps in Italy, Czechoslovakia and Germany. Murray always managed to escape whatever tedium he faced by remembering the mountains and he continued this while captured. But he wanted to take it a stage further and write down his experiences.

He had no paper. One day a parcel arrived from the Red Cross, containing the complete works of Shakespeare and a toilet roll. He reversed the usual functions and *Mountaineering in Scotland* was written on a toilet roll.

The first manuscript was confiscated by the Gestapo, thinking that it was some extremely profound spy document. Undeterred, Murray began the process all over again and, after his release in May 1945, the book was published in 1947. Along with *Undiscovered Scotland*, which he published in 1951, these two books marked Murray, not just as an outstanding mountaineer, but also as a man of some literary worth.

Murray and his companions revolutionised climbing in Scotland, taking it a gigantic leap forward. He and his friends were part of the mountains and loved every minute of their time there. They were true mountaineers in that they loved simply being in the mountains, whether they were sauntering up Munros, clinging to some vertical rock face or chipping their way up an ice gully.

In particular, Murray revitalised and revolutionised Scottish winter climbing. He introduced the short-handled Slater's Pick which makes it easier to cut hand-holds rather than use the long-handled ice axes which were inappropriate for steep climbs. In this respect he can be considered an originator of the current 'front pointing' technique, although others, such as MacInnes, Cunningham and Chouinard, developed it to the current high level of sophistication. The techniques opened up many wonderful climbs to ordinary climbers such as myself.

With the new techniques, he climbed Crowberry Ridge by the Garrick Shelf on Buachaille Etive Mor in 1937, and Deep-Cut Chimney on Stob Coire nam Beith in 1938. Although their difficulty has receded somewhat with modern times, for their day they were outstanding achievements.

Skye had a special place in Murray's heart, as indeed it has for most climbers. His gripping account of ascending the Crack of Doom frightened me off it for a number of years. He was the first to make the greater traverse of the Cuillin Ridge in Skye and, in his later years, he spent many a happy day in Glenbrittle and Sligachan.

Finally, in 1938, just before the War, he cracked Glencoe's Clachaig Gully. I never tire of reading his account of this, and although not now considered difficult, it remains a wonderful expedition.

His prison camp years undoubtedly affected his climbing, and following the War he never quite regained his pre-eminence. Yet, his ascent of Twisting Gully on Stob Coire nan Lochan in 1946 remains a must for every budding 'hardman'. In the early 1950s he was a member of two Himalayan expeditions to Garhwal and Almora in 1950 – and he was deputy leader in Eric Shipton's 1951 Everest reconnaissance. Murray failed to acclimatise at altitude and was not in the 1953 Everest team.

Murray retired to the west coast of Loch Goil to continue his writing and enjoy sailing and climbing with his wife, Anne Burnet Clark. He continued his sterling work with the Mountaineering Council for Scotland, the Countryside Commission for Scotland, the Scottish Countryside Council and the National Trust for Scotland. He occasionally came to dinners of the Scottish Mountaineering Club of which he was Honorary President and where I briefly made his acquaintance.

Bill Murray was one of my heroes. When reading him, I was with him. Along with my father and mother, he was the main force behind my lifelong love of the mountains. He introduced me to a paradise from which I shall not depart. Illness may have broken my ability but the times and the memories linger.

Bill Murray got it right when he said that 'through mountains I have been given not only vivid memories but lasting joys

and friendships more priceless than the accumulations of gold.'
He shared these memories with us and for that I and future
generations will be forever grateful.

William Hutchison Murray, mountaineer and author; born 18
March 1913, died 19 March 1996.

Ministerial Address to Scottish Health
Service Conference
Peebles, Friday 30 May 1997

I am pleased to have this opportunity to address this conference so soon after the election, as it allows me to set out the Government's programme for the Scottish Health Service.

First let me acknowledge the role you all play in helping to manage our health service. As with all the other staff in the Health Service, patients look to you to provide them with effective care, delivered efficiently, and to put their interests first. The dedicated and skilled staff who care for patients also expect you to be enlightened employers, alert and responsive to their concerns.

You will also, I know, recognise your responsibility to give effect to the new Government's policies and to the changes we intend to introduce. The Government has been elected with a clear mandate for change; a mandate to change the Health Service for the better.

We intend to honour the commitments we have made, and to implement the programme which has won the support of people in Scotland. But let me reassure you there will be no big bang, no overnight upheaval. I personally have been through five major upheavals, each one hailed as the last great final solution, only to have it replaced by yet another great final solution.

But change in any organisation is always necessary and we intend to introduce changes in a measured way after they have been tested and fully evaluated. We will pace our changes to take account of the pressures which face the Scottish Health Service day-by-day, and in developing our policies we will listen to patients and to those who serve them.

What will have to change quickly and indeed immediately is thinking. All previous assumptions of where we were going are finished. The internal market is over and I am pleased here today to turn the page and close the chapter on it.

Some things we shall tackle quickly. We have already made a start to honour our pledge to reduce waiting times by switching £10 million from administration to patient care. Two weeks ago I announced our intention to use savings made as a result of cuts in bureaucracy to reduce waiting times and to ensure effective plans are in place to deal with winter peaks in emergency admissions; and I have been impressed with your response in developing plans to achieve these important objectives.

Over the coming months we shall announce further changes, guided by four principles.

We will protect and develop the Scottish Health Service as a public service and will not permit it to be eroded through the privatisation of clinical services. We will focus everyone's efforts on improving the quality of service to patients. We will tackle inequalities in health and in access to health services. We will continue to wage war on waste and bureaucracy.

Labour established the NHS as a public service to bring order to the funding and organisation of health care and to give people a real sense of security that health care would be there when they needed it.

When I had a lung transplant seven years ago, I had many worries. The one worry I did not have was who was going to pay for it.

It is my duty to ensure that this continues and that the Health Service remains free at the point of use, funded through general taxation; and available to all on the basis of need. I want to pass on my parents' legacy to my own children.

We will not permit the Health Service to be eroded by creeping privatisation. But we are prepared to work with the private sector in partnership when that brings benefits to patients. We have inherited a number of proposals to rebuild some of our most prestigious hospitals through the Private Finance Initiative and are reviewing these proposals carefully to make sure they are consistent with our policies and that they do not commit the Health Service to agreements which hinder the proper strategic planning of health care.

We will make sure that any PFI schemes before us exclude clinical services, and we will not permit a repeat of the Stone-haven PFI process. Although the outcome retained clinical services within the Health Service the process placed this principle in jeopardy. Hospital clinical services will be funded and provided by the Scottish Health Service, not by the private sector.

Next let me deal with quality of service. We are making our changes because we believe we can achieve more by working together. Good medicine and effective health care depend on teamwork. This Government believes that collaboration and co-operation will help to improve the quality of services which is the aim of everyone working in the Health Service. As the clinical outcome indicators developed by CRAG show, there is ample evidence of scope for improvement.

There are, across Scotland, variations in outcome and service quality which we must address and we are determined to do so. We must build on some of the excellent clinical audit underway throughout the Scottish Health Service.

The power of collaboration to help tackle these issues is evident in the work underway to implement changes in the organisation of cancer services. This has been characterised by co-operation and co-ordination among Health Boards and Trusts, and among GPs and hospital consultants.

Here is a model which works, and which does so in stark contrast to the destructive power of competition which undermines our capacity to construct the services which I want: seamless, secure and giving patients the continuity of care which is so important, from GP, through the hospital and into rehabilitation in the community.

I want to see the same collaborative approach in your work on the other clinical priorities of mental health and coronary heart disease/stroke.

I have no doubt we must keep these as priorities for the Scottish Health Service. I also have no doubt that primary care, and general medical practitioners in particular, must play an important role in the development of these services.

Inevitably, our search for higher quality will require change. We must replace outdated institutions with modern alternative services in the community for those with mental illness and learning disabilities, recognising that for some people, in-patient care, provided wherever possible in homely settings, will continue to be needed.

We must not rush, as we are sometimes in danger of doing, from inappropriate placement in the hospital to inappropriate placement in the community. The one is as bad as the other.

As work on the acute services review progresses, we will need also to consider changes in the pattern of hospital services. We will want to consult widely on any proposals which emerge, but the Government is prepared to make difficult decisions when the clinical evidence supports the case for change. The public understands this. So did Aneurin Bevan.

When Bevan expressed the preference 'to be kept alive in the efficient if cold altruism of a large hospital than expire in a gush of warm sympathy in a small one', he was acknowledging the need for health services to change and adapt in the face of new needs and new treatment possibilities.

The third of my key principles is equity. Fairness and justice are at the heart of the Scottish ethos; they are also fundamental to the idea of a National Health Service. They have been eroded by policies which have undermined the principle that access to care is determined by clinical need.

Single-practice GP fundholding has opened up a potential for unfairness in securing advantages for some patients at the expense of others, and it involves too much paper and red tape. It distorts the provision of services which affect those outside the practice.

Our intention therefore is to end single-practice fundholding as soon as we can, and to explore new models for the future which are seen by all to be fair and equitable.

I believe that GPs must have a central role in the planning of health services. They have a crucial role in co-ordinating the care of their patients through the complexities of a modern health service and they can help achieve the seamless service which we desire. I am sure that all GPs will welcome the opportunity to work together to be involved in designing and delivering the services which their patients require and which are available on the basis of need.

Addressing inequalities in access to services is part of our strategy for dealing with inequalities in health.

Compared with other parts of the UK, Scotland's health is worse on many indicators. Looking further afield, people in most European nations enjoy a longer life expectancy than is the case of Scotland, and in the key areas of coronary heart disease and cancer Scotland is at or close to the bottom of the league table. These are worrying facts which we shall tackle.

What is more, the national statistics mask deeply worrying variations in health status between social groups and between different parts of our country. Our predecessors may have tried to downplay the existence of these inequalities and to deny the link between them and factors such as poverty, poor housing, and unemployment.

The irrefutable fact is that health is worse in areas where housing is sub-standard, where unemployment is rife, and where poverty abounds. Next month we will be publishing the first Scottish Health Survey which will demonstrate clearly the scale of the problem and enable us to target action where the health need is greatest.

We have promised action to tackle these problems with urgency. Already the Secretary of State has announced a redistribution of spending, from which housing will benefit. Our policies to tackle educational disadvantage, to set a national minimum wage and our welfare-to-work programme will all help. So too, will our plans to ban tobacco advertising, including the use of sports sponsorship as a means of advertising tobacco brands.

But there is much the Health Service can contribute as well, working with others to improve health in our most deprived neighbourhoods.

I expect our planning guidance, which we will issue in the summer, to say more on this. But let me ask you today to respond with energy and initiative to the challenge of tackling health inequalities in Scotland.

You will recognise that this may mean a reassessment of local priorities and resource allocation. At a national level, I have decided that we should look carefully at our arrangements for distributing resources to Health Boards for hospitals, community and family health services, to ensure these fully reflect local population needs and operate as fairly as possible. In particular, I shall want to consider if they make appropriate allowance for factors such as social deprivation and population sparsity.

I am conscious of the scale of the challenge which I have described so far. In part, our capacity to make progress will depend on sweeping away the bureaucracy which has tied the Health Service in red tape.

We are determined to end the current paper chase, to cut down the flow of invoices, to streamline existing management systems, and to replace annual contracts. I have asked the Chief Executive to work urgently with you to ensure that these changes are developed on a sound basis and implemented without delay, and to identify ways in which the new opportunities presented by modern information technology can be harnessed to speed communication and reduce paperwork.

Good managers have always sought to reduce administrative overheads to the minimum, and I want you to seize the opportunity which our commitment to co-operation and collaboration now offers to reduce further the costs of administration, including the costs of financial and personnel management.

The internal market has caused these costs to spiral upwards at the expense of patient care; we must bring this to an end, and I look to the management community to take a lead in making it happen.

Competition has produced unnecessary duplication of many support services and I look to managers as a matter of urgency to collaborate to reduce the costs of those services so as to release funds for patient care.

The Health Service needs good managers and good management; it needs management concentrated on delivering quality care instead of being preoccupied with the wasteful, unproductive administration of an internal market.

I like to think that I am the originator of the much-used phrase about the Health Service being 'over-administered but under-managed'. This came from my lips in 1970 before many of you were around the Health Service. I am on your side. But you must produce significant reductions in your administrative budget and do it soon.

In the Queen's Speech we announced our intention to legislate to replace the internal market. Over the summer we shall be preparing a White Paper which will set out our intentions in detail, describing our plans to develop new models of GP involvement and our plans for trusts and Health Boards.

As I said at the start, we shall adopt a style which is measured, paced and evaluative. But we also intend to take action now to reduce the number of Trusts where the opportunity arises. I know discussions have been taking place amongst some of you about the possibilities for merger. I would expect any reconfiguration of the Trust network to be founded on the development of clinical links between hospitals, and between hospitals and primary care.

We will consider carefully how to take this forward, for I shall want to be sure that it can be achieved with a minimum of disruption and in a manner consistent with our broader aims for the Health Service.

There is another structural issue on which I wish to touch. It is the boundary between health and social care. Some of you may have read my recent article in the BMA News Review in which I express concern that we have not got this boundary right with the result that the seamless service we are trying to provide sometimes breaks down. This is a subject to which we shall be giving careful thought.

In the meantime can I ask you to continue your efforts to work effectively with your partners in social work to ensure that patients receive the services they need, and do not become the subject of a bureaucratic dispute?

The White Paper we shall publish will have more to say on many of the matters I have discussed but our direction of travel is clear. We want the Health Service to be focused on the quality of care to patients; I want a 'same-day' model which minimises the delays in access to care and removes the uncertainty which these delays bring.

I want the patient to be given the date of the Outpatient appointment when they are with their GP. I want the patient to be given the day of their admission when they see the consultant at the Outpatients and I want the patient to have the results of their investigations on the same day that those investigations are carried out. I don't want to hear any more that the patient has been told to come back in a fortnight for the results of their tests.

I also want a Health Service which conducts its business with individuals and the community as openly as possible. The public which funds our Health Service expects it to be open to scrutiny: that is right, and for this reason I have decided that from now on all Trusts – like Health Boards – will be required to hold their meetings in public. Many of you already do so. It is good practice which must be applied throughout the Scottish Health Service.

I conclude by acknowledging the scale of the changes before us. Few Governments have been elected with such a clear mandate to change things for the better. But let me repeat, we shall not pursue change for change's sake.

There will be a Scottish Parliament which will be charged with ensuring that the needs and priorities of Scotland are reflected in the development of our Health Services. This is an exciting time to be Minister for Health in Scotland. There is a lot to do, but I am confident that between us we can make the Scottish Health Service better for patients.

The Origins of My Politics

Reflections written by Sam Galbraith as he was preparing to leave Westminster and Holyrood in 2001.

It was a fine and sunny Saturday at the beginning of May 1997. My battle bus, a splendid vintage Land Rover belonging to my sub-agents David and Hilda Butler, rolled into Kirkintilloch High Street. The crowds were out everywhere and you could hear our tune, 'Things Can Only Get Better'. Locals came up and spoke to me, cheered and shook my hand. A great day! I now knew that we were going to win. After 18 years in opposition, Labour was about to be returned to government. My job of helping to make the Labour Party electable again was over.

How did I get there? Why, people always asked me and still do, was a consultant neurosurgeon in a secure job with a high salary prepared to give up that job security for a reduction in salary?

I was brought up in Greenock, the second of five children. My father was a joiner who, when he was demobbed in 1945 after the war, went to Jordanhill Training College for a year and became a technical teacher. We lived on a peripheral estate in Greenock called Braeside and, although not poor, we never had any of the luxuries of life.

At that time virtually no one where we lived went to university and certainly no one within our extended family did, or would ever have considered it. Most people left school early to work in the shipyards.

My mother left school when she was twelve and suffered for this. Her writing was poor but she was a voracious reader of books. My father was self-taught and widely read and had a keen interest in politics and social justice. There were lots and lots of books in our house and we were regular visitors to the library.

Even from my earliest days I remember my Mum and Dad mentioning that we would go to university and I was taken to see the great building up the hill in Glasgow. I even remember my father's words: 'If you stick in at school, Samuel, one day you'll come here and study medicine.'

And so I did. But that was only after I had seen all my schoolmates, who were really clever, follow the accepted trend and leave school at 15 for the yards. They were clever individuals but in Greenock at that time very few went to university. When I left school, only a handful of us moved on to university. We were part of the elite 2 per cent.

It was because of this background that I used to get angry when I would hear all the so-called 'socialists' bleating on about how tuition fees and the graduate tax would stop 'working-class' kids going to university. What rubbish! They didn't realise that under the system they wanted to return to – the one that I was brought up under, with fees paid and bursaries – working-class kids didn't go to university. It was only an elite 2 per cent. Reintroducing that system would cut the numbers again and it would be the working-class kids who would lose out again. The few of us that did go to university went on the backs of all the other working-class kids. They paid for us to go by not going themselves.

I was off to be a doctor. My parents wanted me to go to the mission fields. It would be a great advantage if I went there as a doctor. I had a very strict religious upbringing in the Elim Church, which is a Presbyterian Pentecostal organisation. I became an atheist but my desire to become a doctor remained. My parents never interfered.

In the morning I would be off to Glasgow University from my home in Greenock. As I got on the bus one cold morning I sat down with the men in their boiler suits, previous classmates of mine. I got off the bus into a warm train, and looking out from my comfortable seat I could see the shipyards. There were my classmates working outside on the ships in freezing, driving sleet while I was off to the university. It wasn't fair and it wasn't right and I was determined that one day I would come back to try to ensure that all of these people also had the opportunities that I had.

At university I was an anarchist. I had had enough of the establishment, politics and clubs; they all needed tearing down and rebuilt if we were to make progress. The slogans slipped easily off my tongue. We had our vision of the ideal society and it was round the corner. These were the days of dreams.

But, as always, life's experience gradually impinges on you and gets the upper hand. As the facts change, or at least as we perceive them to change, so too do we. I would have to start joining the political establishment, as it was the only way to bring about the changes to society I wanted.

In due course I joined the Labour Party, whereupon I realised that the Labour Party had huge problems and had to be changed. It was concerned only with the interests of the producers: the teachers, the doctors, the trade unions. Those using the service, if they were considered at all, were of secondary importance. We were detached from the life of the majority of people by being more interested in political dogma than social justice. By 1983, we were walking a road to extinction and would never win an election unless we started appealing to the middle class.

I remember one Party member saying after the '87 election that although we'd lost we still had our principles. Much good that was, especially to all these people we were out to help. 'By their deeds ye shall know them.' (*Matthew* 7, 16). I am not so much concerned with what people claim to be, rather how they behave. Particularly in Scotland, Labour remains too connected to the producer interest rather than the people who depend upon public services. The middle class has only loaned us its vote, and any attempt to go back to the bad old days would be a disaster.

In the late 1970s and early '80s I was becoming politically more and more active. I was attending meetings and taking part in demonstrations, when along came a strike by health workers. I had seen two previous ones and had been a doctor at the time. I knew all the press propaganda about how they were killing patients and threatening patients' lives. I knew this to be complete rubbish as I worked in the National Health Service and knew the reality of what was happening. I was determined that in this struggle I would help the health workers to obtain a better wage settlement.

They did well and in fact the Tories doubled the offer, albeit only from 1 to 2 per cent. I had never expected the Tories would offer more money, and when they did I thought the unions would settle. They didn't and the strike gradually petered out. It was then I began to realise how poor some of the trade union leaders were, leading their members into cul-de-sacs. My activities on behalf of the health workers brought me some notoriety and I was asked to consider whether or not I would stand for Parliament. I always knew that one day this would happen and I had no intention of being a neurosurgeon until I was 65. But I wasn't quite ready at that stage. The pressure from the Party nevertheless increased. We were third in the opinion polls and facing extinction.

The initial approach came from Hillhead, the constituency in which I lived. Although I would have liked to fight it, the sitting member was Roy Jenkins and I felt I was too inexperienced to stand against him and would be crucified at public meetings.

I was then approached by the Strathkelvin and Bearsden constituency and I was more than interested. The Labour Party was third, well behind the Tories and the Liberals, and it would be a hard seat to win. But if we were to win it, we would be in power. My selection was unusual in that I missed all the meetings because I was climbing in the Himalayas. Labour's Scottish organiser at the time was Jimmy Allison who, in his usual splendid manner, smashed down any objections that were raised concerning my absence. And so without much ado I was the prospective parliamentary candidate and launched into the fray. In 1987 I was then elected the Labour Member of Parliament for Strathkelvin and Bearsden.

My journey to parliamentarian was, I think, the right way. I am very much opposed to career politicians who go to university or up through trade unions with the sole aim of going to Parliament. Many nowadays have never had a real job, and certainly never a job outside politics. They then are elected at a young age with little experience in life and unable to make the necessary judgements. Politicians should be asked by the community to stand for them, not impose themselves on the community. Once elected, they should necessarily limit their time and make way for others. It ought not to be a job for life.

My training as a surgeon was excellent preparation for being a politician. As a surgeon you learn to take decisions, tough decisions, indeed decisions that sometimes you wish you could take the opposite way, but still you have to take them. Having taken them, you have to see them through and accept responsibility – good training for politicians.

Politics is an honourable and laudable profession. Much is said about politicians and they are abused, laughed at, condemned and treated with contempt, and most of it is completely unjustified. Yes, there are some characters who fall below high standards, but this must not be used to tar the others. Most politicians are honourable and work extremely hard for other people. They give up large salaries and secure jobs and their families pay a dreadful price. They don't deserve the abuse they get. We should be careful about how we treat them, otherwise there is a danger of developing politicians who will make the myths come true.

In February 1987 Glenys Kinnock was coming to visit my constituency in the lead-up to the June election. I had not been feeling all that well for a few days but, as always, had continued on. I had a bit of a 'flu but nevertheless I struggled through Glenys's visit which was great fun. When I left her I drove to the Cairngorms to go skiing, but could only make it to lunchtime on the slopes on the Saturday. I had never felt so bad. I went back to the hotel, went straight to bed and didn't eat. I started coughing up quite a large amount of blood. I had noticed this on the mountain when I was skiing and thought it was just irritation from my excess coughing.

I went back to work on Monday morning feeling really lousy. My colleagues forced me to have a chest X-ray and there were signs of pneumonia. I went to see my physician and he prescribed an antibiotic. I went back to see him a week later, why I know not, because as far as I was concerned I had swallowed the tablets and kept working and that ought to have been the end of it. The moment I sat down I knew there was something different. The doctor explained that it wasn't just pneumonia, but I had the disease called fibrosing alveolitis. I knew that was death in two to three years.

I am surprised looking back that I was so untouched by the information. I just accepted it. I had three years left to live. What should I do? At that time I wasn't keen on a transplant, and it had always been my intention, therefore, that if I ever had a fatal disease I would retire to the Highlands with a bottle of malt and the *Guardian*. However I just wasn't ready to give up at this stage. I never felt angry but I remember once I felt very jealous seeing a grandfather with his young grandchildren, something that was not going to be open to me.

With that diagnosis I finally convinced myself that I really was feeling lousy and very sick and that it was in no one's interests for me to keep working. I took a couple of weeks off and went up through my beloved Highlands and to the Western Isles where I stayed at Brian and Joni Wilson's house.

I realised I would have to make the decision about standing for election. Would I be fit enough, would I be able to handle Parliament, would I be betraying all those who had supported me if I died three years into my first term? I never asked for any advice but I talked to people, not about me or my position but about politics. The more I talked, the more I realised that I had to stand. As I had only three years left to live this would be my only chance to try and fulfil the promise I had made to myself as I sat in the warm train on my way to the University, passing my schoolmates who were freezing cold up on the sides of the ships in the Greenock yards.

With the fantastic support of my Constituency Party, I fought and won the campaign. It was a stunning victory and the finest campaign I have ever been involved in – literally hundreds of helpers and 85 per cent of the constituency was canvassed. To paraphrase George Brown: 'Brothers, we were on our way.'

Medical Publications and Interviews

Peer-reviewed Medical Publications

Fragmentation of cardiac myofibrils after therapeutic starvation.
Galbraith, S.L. *Lancet.* 1(7607):1215–6, 1969.

The mesangium of the renal glomerulus.
Galbraith, S.L. *Scottish Medical Journal.* 16(10):428–37, 1971.

Age-distribution of extradural haemorrhage without skull fracture.
Galbraith, S.L. *Lancet.* 1(7814):1217–8, 1973.

Acute impairment of brain function-2. Observation record chart.
Teasdale, G., Galbraith, S., Clark K. *Nursing Times.* 71(25):972–3, 1975.

Acute traumatic intracranial haematoma without skull fracture.
Galbraith, S., Smith, J. *Lancet.* 1(7958):501–3, 1976.

Computerised tomography of acute traumatic intracranial haematoma: reliability of neurosurgeon's interpretations.
Galbraith, S., Teasdale, G., Blaiklock, C. *British Medical Journal.* 2(6048):1371–3, 1976.

Misdiagnosis and delayed diagnosis in intracranial haematoma.
Galbraith, S. *British Medical Journal.* 1(6023):1438–9, 1976.

The relationship between alcohol and head injury and its effect on the conscious level.
Galbraith, S., Murray, W.R., Patel, A.R., Knill-Jones, R. *British Journal of Surgery.* 63(2):128–30, 1976.

Penetrating airgun injuries of the head.
Shaw, M.D., Galbraith, S. *British Journal of Surgery.* 64(3):221–4, 1977.

Alcohol and head injury.
Patel, A.R., Jennett, B., Galbraith, S. *Lancet.* 1(8026):1369–70, 1977.

Severe head injuries in three countries.
Jennett, B., Teasdale, G., Galbraith, S., Pickard, J., Grant, H., Braakman, R., Avezaat, C., Maas, A., Minderhoud, J., Vecht, C.J., Heiden, J., Small, R., Caton, W., Kurze, T. *Journal of Neurology, Neurosurgery and Psychiatry.* 40(3):291–8, 1977.

Head injury admissions to a teaching hospital.
Galbraith, S., Murray, W.R., Patel, A.R. *Scottish Medical Journal.* 22(2):129–32, 1977.

The 'no lose' philosophy in medicine.
Galbraith, S. *Journal of Medical Ethics.* 4(2):61–3, 1978.

Categories of axons in mammalian rami communicantes. Part II.
Coggeshall, R.E., Galbraith, S.L. *Journal of Comparative Neurology.* 181(2):349–59, 1978.

The afferent fibres of the sympathetic nervous system.
Galbraith, S. *Acta Neurochirurgica – Supplementum.* 28(2):613–5, 1979.

Prognosis in patients with severe head injury.
Jennett, B., Teasdale, G., Galbraith, S., Braakman, R., Avezaat, C., Minderhoud, J., Heiden, J., Kurze, T., Murray, G.,
Parker, L. *Acta Neurochirurgica – Supplementum.* 28(1):149–52,
1979.

Management of patients with subarachnoid haemorrhage.
Galbraith, S.L. *Nursing Times.* 75(43)1852–4, 1979.

Infection after depressed fracture in the West of Scotland.
Sande, G.M., Galbraith, S.L., McLatchie, G. *Scottish Medical
Journal.* 25(3):227–9, 1980.

Electron-microscopic study of the synapses of the cerebral
cortex in man.
Galbraith, S. *Acta Anatomica.* 107(1):46–51, 1980.

Management of traumatic intracranial haematoma.
Teasdale, G., Galbraith, S., Murray, L., Ward, P., Gentleman,
D., McKean, M. *British Medical Journal Clinical Research Ed.*
285(6356):1695–7, 1982.

Analysis of the cerebrospinal fluid pulse wave in intracranial
pressure.
Cardoso, E.R., Rowan, J.O., Galbraith, S. *Journal of Neurosurgery.* 59(5):817–21, 1983.

An Introduction to Neurosurgery (Third Edition).
Jennett, B., Galbraith, S. William Heinemann, London 1983
[Book].

CT scan in severe diffuse head injury: physiological and clinical correlations.
Teasdale, E., Cardoso, E., Galbraith, S., Teasdale, G. *Journal of Neurology, Neurosurgery and Psychiatry.* 47(6):600–3, 1984.

Irritability.
Galbraith, S. *British Medical Journal Clinical Research Edition.* 291(1668–9), 1985. [Editorial]

Dementia due to meningioma: outcome after surgical removal.
Chee, C.P., David, A., Galbraith, S., Gillham, R. *Surgical Neurology.* 23(4):414–6, 1985.

Posttraumatic hydrocephalus – a retrospective review.
Cardoso, E.R., Galbraith, S. *Surgical Neurology.* 23(3):261–4, 1985.

Hemimegalencephaly – a case for hemispherectomy?
King, M., Stephenson, J.B., Ziervogel, M., Doyle, D., Galbraith, S. *Neuropediatrics.*16 (1):46–55, 1985.

The effect of mannitol on cerebral white matter water content.
Nath, F., Galbraith, S. *Journal of Neurosurgery.* 65(1):41–3, 1986.

Necropsy study of mountaineering accidents in Scotland.
Reid, W.A., Doyle, D., Richmond, H.G., Galbraith, S.L. *Journal of Clinical Pathology.* 39(11):1217–20, 1986.

The significance of traumatic haematoma in the region of the basal ganglia.
Macpherson, P., Teasdale, E., Dhaker, S., Allerdyce, G., Galbraith, S. *Journal of Neurology, Neurosurgery and Psychiatry.* 49(1):29–34, 1986.

A neuropsychological study of active amateur boxers.
Books, N., Kupshik, G., Wilson, L., Galbraith, S., Ward, R.
Journal of Neurology, Neurosurgery and Psychiatry. 50(8):997–
1000, 1987.

Clinical neurological examination, neuropsychology, electroen-
cephalography and computed tomographic head scanning in
active amateur boxers.
McLatchie, G., Brooks, N., Galbraith S., Hutchins, J.S.,
Wilson, L., Melville, I., Teasdale, E. *Journal of Neurology,
Neurosurgery and Psychiatry.* 50(1):96–9, 1987.

Magnetic resonance imaging in the management of resistant
focal epilepsy: pathological case report and experience of 12 cases.
Grant, R., Hadley, D.M., Condon, B., Doyle, D., Patterson, J.,
Bone, I., Galbraith, S.L., Teasdale, G.M. *Journal of Neurology,
Neurosurgery and Psychiatry.* 50(11):1529–32, 1987.

Carotid traumatic aneurysm treated by detachable balloon.
Crandon, I.W., Teasdale, E., Galbraith, S.L., Hadley, D.M.
British Journal of Neurosurgery. 2(4):507–11, 1988.

The management outcome of patients with a ruptured poste-
rior circulation aneurysm.
Lang, D.A., Galbraith, S.L. *Acta Neurochirurgica.* 125(1–4):9–
14, 1993.

Therapeutic potential of endothelin receptor antagonists in
experimental stroke.
Patel, T.R., Galbraith, S.L., McAuley, M.A. Doherty, A.M.,
Graham, D.I., McCulloch, J. *Journal of Cardiovascular Phar-
macology.* 26 Suppl 3:S412–5, 1995.

Endothelin receptor antagonist increases cerebral perfusion and reduces ischaemic damage in feline focal cerebral ischaemia.
Patel, T.R., Galbraith, S., Graham, D.I., Hallak, H., Doherty, A.M., McCulloch, J. *Journal of Cerebral Blood Flow and Metabolism.* 16(5):950–8, 1996.

Endothelin-mediated vascular tone following focal cerebral ischaemia in the cat.
Patel, T.R., Galbraith, S., McAuley, M.A., McCulloch, J. *Journal of Cerebral Blood Flow and Metabolism.* 16(4):679–87, 1996.

Endothelin-B receptors in cerebral resistance arterioles and their functional significance after focal cerebral ischemia in cats.
Touzani, O., Galbraith, S., McAuley, M.A., McCulloch, J. *Journal of Cerebral Blood Flow and Metabolism.* 17(11):1157–65, 1997.

The relationship between glutamate release and cerebral blood flow after focal cerebral ischaemia in the cat: effect of pretreatment with enadoline (a kappa receptor agonist).
MacKay, K.B., Patel, T.R., Galbraith, S.L., Woodruff, G.N., McCulloch, J. *Brain Research.* 712(2):329–34, 1996 Mar 18.

Working together.
Galbraith, S. *Nursing Standard.* 13(27):22, 1999 Mar 24–30.

Does health care improve health?
Craig, N., Wright, B., Hanlon, P., Galbraith, S. *Journal of Health Services and Research Policy.* 11(1):1–2, 2006.

Interviews

There's a doctor in the house. Interview by Rebecca Coombes. Galbraith, S. *Nursing Times.* 94(15):15, 1998.

A recording of an interview conducted by Mr Iain Macintyre and Mr D. Wright is held at the Royal College of Surgeons of Edinburgh: Interview with Sam Galbraith, 2007. Surgeons' Hall Museum video archive, ED.CS.2015.11.